*The Essential Guide
to the Hottest Supplements
for Wellness and Longevity*

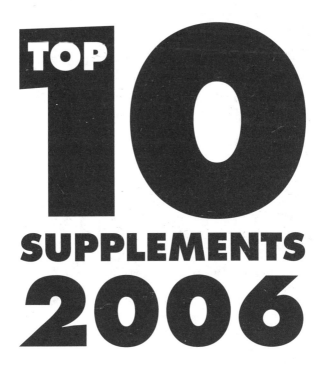

TOP

10

SUPPLEMENTS

2006

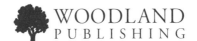

WOODLAND
PUBLISHING

Copyright © 2006 by Woodland Publishing

A cataloging-in-publication record for this book is available from the Library of Congress.

For ordering information, contact:
Woodland Publishing, 448 E 800 North, Orem, UT 84097
(800) 777-2665

Note: The information contained in this book is for educational purposes only and is not recommended as a means of diagnosing or treating an illness. All matters concerning mental and physical health should be supervised by a health practitioner knowledgable in treating that particular condition. Neither the publisher nor the authors directly or indirectly dispenses medical advice, nor do they prescribe any remedies or assume any responsibility for those who choose to treat themselves.

ISBN 1-58054-415-0

Printed in the United States of America
1   2   3   4   5   6   7   8   9   10

Please visit our website:
www.woodlandpublishing.com

Açai Berry

Cinnamon

Conjugated Linoleic Acid

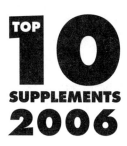

TOP 10 SUPPLEMENTS 2006

Cranberry

Hoodia

Hyaluronic Acid

Mango

Nattokinase

Omega-3 Fatty Acids

Wolfberry

CONTENTS

INTRODUCTION

Today more than 100 million Americans are taking some sort of nutritional supplement to prevent or treat disease and promote overall wellness and longevity. These supplements range from vitamins and minerals to homeopathic remedies, herbs, antioxidants, and other bioactive compounds.

With an influx of thousands of new supplements each year, accompanied by a barrage of advice, conflicting expert opinions, and promises of miraculous results, the editors of Woodland Publishing felt a book was needed that would focus on the ten hottest supplements—those that are new to the market and those that demonstrate recently discovered beneficial properties.

The supplements discussed in this book contain nutrients that are crucial for the proper functioning of the human body. They provide wide-ranging benefits and are involved in varied and vital bodily functions. Of course, you could certainly educate yourself about the benefits of other supplements not discussed here, and we encourage you to do so. But for those who are simply left bewildered and overwhelmed by the flood of new supplements, over-hyped products, and contradictory advice, this book is your best bet to finding and benefiting from the hottest supplements today.

THE TOP 10

Açai Berry

From deep in the Amazon rain forest comes the sweet, deep-purple açai berry. With remarkable antioxidant properties, the açai berry shows promise in helping to prevent inflammation, heart disease, and reduce the signs of aging.

Cinnamon

The old familiar kitchen standby is demonstrating some remarkable properties in recent research. A water-soluble polyphenol in cinnamon can help lower blood sugar levels in diabetics, pre-diabetics, and others with blood sugar problems. Plus, cinnamon has antibacterial and antifungal properties and can help relieve intestinal distress, prevent colds and flu, and lower blood cholesterol.

Conjugated Linoleic Acid

An essential fatty acid that was first identified in the 1970s, CLA has demonstrated powerful anticancer potential, can help prevent the clogging of arteries, and can help reduce body fat while building lean muscle tissue.

Cranberry

This Thanksgiving staple—the most antioxidant-rich common fruit—can provide benefits in preventing heart disease, strokes, and cancer. Cranberries also possess remarkable properties that prevent the adherence of harmful microbes in the urinary tract, and, potentially, other areas of the body.

Hoodia

From Africa's Kalahari desert comes an exotic succulent that Bushmen have used for thousands of years to slake their thirst and curb their appetites. Hoodia has been demonstrated in clinical studies to work as a potent appetite suppressant for those who are struggling with obesity and excess weight.

Hyaluronic Acid

A major component in all connective tissue in the body, hyaluronic acid binds water molecules to cells and tissues. This enables the smooth functioning of connective tissue, especially in joints. As we age, hyaluronic acid production decreases and the fluids surrounding our joints start to "dry up," contributing to osteoarthritis. Recent studies indicate that injections and oral supplemention of hyaluronic acid reduces the pain and suffering of osteoarthritis.

Mangosteen

With baby boomers hitting their fifties, many are turning to antioxidants to stay healthy and prevent disease. Drinking mangosteen juice or taking mangosteen pericarp capsules can give us a powerhouse of tannins, catechins, and xanthones to arm our body with enough antioxidants to help minimize the free radicals waging war against our health.

Nattokinase

Though it's stinky and slimy in its natural state, the fermented soy product nattokinase has demonstrated some pretty remarkable health-promoting qualities in clinical research. Chief among them is nattokinase's ability to improve circulatory health through its blood-thinning and anticlotting properties. With heart disease and stroke the number-one and number-three killers in the United States, nattokinase may prove to be a significant addition to the arsenal of disease-preventing supplements now available.

Omega-3 Fatty Acids

Research into the health-promoting effects of omega-3s is ongoing, but enough studies have demonstrated how crucial these essential fatty acids are. Whether you feast on wild Alaskan salmon, sprinkle ground flax seeds on your cereal, or take one of the many fish oil capsules available, you're taking an important step toward ensuring your overall health and well-being.

Wolfberry

The wolfberry, ancient China's "national treasure" that has bestowed youth and vigor on generations of Chinese, is now available as modern America's most potent anti-oxidant food. Numerous clinical studies have demonstrated that the wolfberry can play a significant role in preventing free radical damage and oxidative stress, supporting a healthy immune system, improving vision, and assisting in maintaining healthy blood sugar levels.

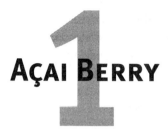AÇAI BERRY

If you traveled deep into the Amazon rain forests of Brazil, you would find thousands of miles of Amazon palm trees. And high in the tops of these trees grow berries called açai (*Enterpe oleracea*). Pronounced AH-sigh-EE, these deep-purple berries resemble small marbles and have an unusual taste of sweet berry with just a hint of chocolate. While connoisseurs say açai has a taste similar to chocolate-covered cherries—health experts say it has almost as many nutrients as most multivitamins.

The açai berry, a small, almost perfectly round, dark-purple fruit grows on the Brazilian wild palmberry tree, where natives have benefited from its powerful antioxidants for hundreds of years. Açai is traditionally puréed and served as a sauce. Brazilians also use the berry in drinks or in ice cream or ice smoothies sold on the street. The delicious açai drinks are especially popular in the beach resorts of Brazil.

Açai, used for hundreds of years by native Brazilians for its various health benefits, is just now beginning to take center stage in the Western world. But now it's gaining popularity in the United States—especially on the West Coast, where it's commonly used in juice bars as a tasty, healthy addition to popular smoothie recipes.

The taste certainly attracts the modern consumer, but it's the amazing health properties of the açai berry that are starting to get the attention of the health industry. Açai is packed with potent antioxidants. The main sources of antioxidants in açai are anthocyanins, which give the berry its purple color. Açai contains ten to thirty-three times the amount of anthocyanins found in red wine. More than just simply an antioxidant fruit, açai contains valuable amino acids, unsaturated fats, and phytosterols and offers numerous health benefits for the entire body.

Nicholas Perricone, author of *The Perricone Promise* and *The Perricone Prescription*, recently touted the benefits of açai on the *Oprah Winfrey Show*, naming it one of "Ten Superfoods for Age-Defying Beauty."

Because açai has so many powerful health benefits, let's discuss each one individually.

Antioxidants

One of the most serious problems facing modern human health is oxidative stress. Oxidative stress means there aren't enough antioxidants in your body to control the free radical population. Oxidative stress, caused by free radicals wreaking havoc inside your body, is making you age every minute of every day. Your best tool to combat the aging process is antioxidant support. Antioxidants are substances that neutralize free radicals and stop their destructive assault on the cells of the body. Free radicals are so damaging because they're unbalanced. They lack a shared electron. An antioxidant molecule donates one of its own electrons to the rogue free radical and restores balance. Antioxidants also work together with your body to repair the harm caused by free radicals.

The Nuts and Bolts of Antioxidants

Antioxidants exist within your body and also within nature. Some of the more well-known antioxidants include vitamin C, vitamin E, selenium, and the carotenoids. Research has also uncovered high antioxidant values in certain fruits and vegetables, including berries, *especially açai berries*. Sales of antioxidant supplements have been on the rise in recent years, with revenues increasing 6 percent in 2003 to $2.7 billion worldwide, as reported by the *Nutrition Business Journal*. Many of these supplements can help, but few are as potent and offer as many other, non-antioxidant, benefits as açai.

Antioxidants support the body in many different ways:
- Promote cardiovascular and circulatory health
- Control excessive inflammation
- Maintain healthy cholesterol levels
- Promote digestive system health
- Boost the immune system
- Reduce the signs of aging

Anthocyanins

Anthocyanins are some of the most powerful antioxidants. Their potency and health value are especially visible in the French diet. You may have heard of the "French paradox," in which the people of France eat a high-fat diet and have an unhealthy lifestyle common in Western society, but the incidence of cardiovascular disease is lower in France than in the United States and the United Kingdom.

One reason may be the large amounts of red wine they consume. Red wine is made from grapes with very high levels of anthocyanins. Experts believe these anthocyanins somehow mitigate the effects of high-fat diets and cigarette smoking. Anthocyanins are also shown in studies to improve the symptoms of many age-related diseases.

Anthocyanins have a unique chemical structure, making them six to eight times more potent than vitamin C. According to intense research, açai contains the most highly concentrated forms of anthocyanins now known. The anthocyanin content in a small amount of açai was recently tested against a glass of red wine. The results showed that açai contains three-and-a-half times more anthocyanins than one glass of red wine.

ORAC Value

In the past thirty years, a procedure has been developed, tested repeatedly, and perfected to help determine the who's who list of antioxidants. The Oxygen Radical Absorbance Capacity, often referred to as the ORAC value, measures the total antioxidant value of foods and other chemical substances. The antioxidant value is defined as the ability of a compound to reduce the amount of free radicals within the body. The higher the ORAC value, the more antioxidant value that particular substance carries. The açai berry has one of the highest ORAC values of any naturally occurring substance—plant or animal based.

In recent U.S. Agricultural Research Service studies on foods with high ORAC values, scientists found that eating high-ORAC foods like açai:

- Raised the antioxidant power of human blood 10 to 25 percent
- Prevented some loss of long-term memory and learning ability in middle-aged rats
- Maintained the ability of brain cells in middle-aged rats to respond to a chemical stimulus—a function that normally decreases with age
- Protected rats' capillaries against oxygen damage

"If these findings are borne out in further research, young and middle-aged people may be able to reduce risk of diseases of aging—including senility—simply by adding high-ORAC foods to their diets," said ARS administrator Floyd P. Horn.

The value of antioxidants is now firmly based in scientific fact. Their ability to scavenge free radicals and reverse the effects of premature aging simply cannot be ignored. With oxidative stress occurring everywhere in your body, antioxidants provide real support and real solutions to turn back the clock and help you feel younger than you actually are.

Joe Barron, president of the Baseline of Health Foundation and a world leader on health and nutrition, says the following about the benefits of açai:

> Açai is a particularly potent source of anthocyanins, the powerful class of antioxidants that helps prevent blood clots, improves circulation, relaxes blood vessels, prevents atherosclerosis and combats cancer. In addition, açai is also a source of oleic acid, which in addition to promoting heart health blocks the action of a cancer-causing oncogene found in about 30 percent of breast cancer patients.

Açai is one of the most potent antioxidant fruits known to humankind. Based on this fact alone, açai should have a place in any supplement program. But don't forget, there are several other impressive benefits in this little chocolate-flavored berry.

Açai's antioxidant content leaves other fruits in the dust:
- 50 times greater than mangoes
- 3 time greater than blueberries
- 2 times greater than pomegranates
- 10 to 33 times greater than red wine grapes

Unsaturated Fats

Açai contains healthy fats that are necessary for growth, nutrition, and development. There are two types of fat, saturated and unsaturated. Saturated fats, although needed in small amounts by the body, should be largely avoided. Unsaturated fats are the so-called good fats that the body requires on a daily basis. These fats contain crucial building blocks of information for the heart, circulatory system, brain, and skin. The three types of unsaturated fats are omega-3, omega-6, and omega-9.

Açai provides two important and often hard to get unsaturated fats, omega-6 (linolcic acid) and omega-9 (oleic acid). Research shows that these fatty acids play an important role in maintaining healthy cholesterol levels. Omega-9 fatty acids help lower LDL (harmful cholesterol) while maintaining HDL (beneficial cholesterol) levels. Omega-6 essential fatty acids have also been found to lower LDL cholesterol.

CALCIUM

Calcium is one of the most well-known nutrients necessary to health, but what many people don't know is that a little berry from Brazil is one of the richest sources of calcium in the world. Puréed açai contains more calcium per ounce than milk. For a person in need of antioxidant support and calcium supplementation, açai is a perfect and delicious option.

AMINO ACIDS

Amino acids are molecules that make up proteins and carry out important functions throughout the body. They build cells, repair tissue, and form antibodies to fight invading germs. Açai contains two amino acids, methionine and lysine. Methionine promotes healthy cholesterol levels, reduces liver fat, protects the kidneys, and promotes hair growth. Lysine helps your body absorb calcium, promotes healthy bone cartilage and connective tissue, and plays a role in the production of antibodies, hormones, and enzymes.

Phytosterols

Phytosterols, also referred to as plant sterols, are natural substances that are found in the cells and membranes of plants. Açai contains valuable phytosterols such as beta-sitosterol. These sterols provide numerous benefits to the human body, including the reduction of harmful cholesterol. Researchers have also studied the effects of sterols with BPH (benign prostate hyperplasia) and have found them to be an effective treatment for the condition. Beta-sitosterol has been investigated for its use in supporting the immune system, particularly immune weakness that results from physical stress placed on the body.

Carbohydrates for Increased Energy

Açai is also rich in carbohydrates, which can provide your body with a much-needed extra boost of energy to feel better and experience more vitality throughout the day, every day.

Other Nutrients

Açai is also rich in vitamins C and E, iron, manganese, chromium, copper, and boron. The açai berry truly is like a multivitamin in the form of a fruit.

Açai and Your Health

The nutrients described above have some real and important effects on your health. Let's discuss some of the conditions that these nutrients can affect.

Digestive Support and Cancer Prevention

Açai is an excellent source of fiber. Your doctor has probably mentioned to you a number of times that a high-fiber diet can provide protection against cancer, diabetes, heart disease, and obesity. But most of us only get about half the fiber we need each day. There are two types of fiber, soluble and insoluble. Soluble fiber is important for reducing levels of blood cholesterol within the body, and recent research also shows that insoluble fiber may help reduce the risk of contracting certain kinds of cancer.

Inflammation

Inflammation is one of the most serious problems facing us today. Many health experts believe that inflammation may very well be the cause of most serious diseases. Inflammation occurs either when the body has been injured or when the body attacks itself in response to a perceived injury, in what are known as autoimmune disorders. Açai's powerful antioxidants neutralize enzymes that attack connective tissues, alleviating inflammation and regulating the body's response to invaders.

Nervous System Support

Açai's potent antioxidants prevent tyrosine nitration. That sounds like so much science-speak, but what it means is pretty simple and significant. Tyrosine nitration is present in many neurological diseases, and since anthocyanin antioxidants found in açai prevent tyrosine nitration, they may well protect against many neurological diseases.

Blood Vessels

Anthocyanins protect the endothelial cells that make up the surface of blood-vessel walls by countering free radicals that, if left alone, would attack looking for an electron to complete their molecular structures. Each attack damages endothelial cells, causing inflammation, which eventually leads to the buildup of plaque. We all know that plaque on the walls of your blood vessels inevitably causes cardiovascular disease.

Diabetes

One of the severest complications of diabetes is retinopathy, which is the result of the body's attempts to repair damaged capillaries. In repairing this damage, the body overproduces abnormal proteins, which cause retinopathy. Anthocyanins protect against this capillary damage by preventing free radical damage to the circulatory system, from the largest artery to the tiniest microcapillary.

Other Uses

Recent studies show that, in addition to the health benefits listed above, açai may help protect against prostate
disorders like benign prostatic hyperplasia and prostatitis.
Other studies show that açai may improve lipoprotein
metabolism, helping our bodies process fats more effi-
ciently. Another study shows that it bolsters the activity of
the immune system. Natives who have eaten açai for centuries consider it to be a powerful aphrodisiac. Brazilians
often use açai with guaraná extract, a popular natural
substance taken from a seed native to Brazil that is ground
into powder. The combination acts as a powerful caffeine-
like stimulant. Açai is also a dietary staple of Brazilian
athletes.

USING AÇAI

The açai berry spoils quite easily, and since it's grown only
in the Amazon at the current time, it has been a little hard
to find in the United States. But nutritional supplement
manufacturers are starting to bring production online,
and açai should now be readily available in health food
stores or from direct marketers.

According to Joe Barron, "And even if it were [readily
available], it's not really a user-friendly fruit. Only the skin
has flavor and health value—which means your only real
option is finding either açai juice or frozen pulp in a health
food store." Your best bet is probably to find a good juice,
pulp, or extract supplement from a reputable supplement

company. If you go out and buy the raw berries, you're not going to get much out of them. The berries themselves have little fruit. Each berry is about 20 percent fruit and 80 percent pit. You'll get more value and benefit from a juice or supplement form manufactured by a supplement company—just make sure to buy from a company with the best manufacturing practices in place. For example, açai is more valuable the quicker it is taken from harvesting to processing.

WHY IT'S HOT!

As modern science continues to research and better understand the role of oxidative stress in the aging process and the growth of cancer cells, potent antioxidants like açai berries offer a real option with potentially important benefits for those who want to take control of their health. Also, as inflammation is increasingly recognized as a possible underlying cause of heart disease and many other serious conditions, consuming a variety of high-ORAC foods like açai berries may well be just what the doctor ordered.

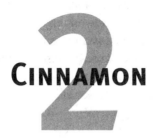

CINNAMON

What scent brings comfort and peace like cinnamon? From cinnamon rolls to apple pie, cinnamon is a commonly used spice not only in the United States, but all around the globe.

HISTORY OF CINNAMON

Found in ancient Chinese texts on herbal medicines dating back about four thousand years, cinnamon has been used for a variety of purposes including medicinal, culinary, and practical. As one of the oldest remedies in traditional Chinese medicine, cinnamon has been used to treat a variety of ailments, including diarrhea, influenza, and parasitic worms.

Not as readily accessible as it is today, cinnamon was a prized spice that reflected great power and prestige upon its possessor. During the explorations of the fifteenth and sixteenth centuries, it was not only the most sought-after spice, but the reason that many explorations were launched in the first place.

The best cinnamon is found in its birthplace of Sri Lanka (formerly Ceylon). A close cousin to cinnamon, cassia, is frequently mistaken for cinnamon and actually tends to reign in the market in North America. We'll talk about the difference between cinnamon and cassia later in this chapter.

In Egypt, cinnamon was valued above gold—which isn't saying a whole lot since gold was plentiful and Egyptians featured it prominently in their decorating and ornamentation. Cinnamon was used as a flavor in drinks and also as a preservative in their embalming process.

In 65 A.D., Roman emperor Nero placed a year's supply of cinnamon on the funeral pyre of his wife, Poppaea Sabina, which was his way of expressing how deeply he would miss her.

During the Black Death period of the bubonic plague, sponges were soaked in cinnamon and cloves and placed in sick rooms. Also at this time in Europe, cinnamon featured heavily in recipes. Most meals were cooked in one pot, including both meat and fruit, and cinnamon helped better combine the sweet and savory flavors in the meal.

Also at that time cinnamon was used as a preservative for meat, which accounts for its heavy use in dishes including chicken and lamb in the Middle East and North Africa.

As early as 2,000 B.C., cinnamon was imported to Egypt from China. The cinnamon trade during the Middle Ages still followed essentially the same route, but passed through many hands. Arab traders brought it into Egypt, where it was bought by Italian traders who kept a close grip on the cinnamon trade in Europe.

By the end of the fifteenth century, Portuguese traders discovered Ceylon and monopolized the trade of Ceylon cinnamon for over one hundred years by building a fort on the island.

In the mid–seventeenth century, Dutch traders expelled the Portuguese, took control of all the factories, and established a trading post. In the process of perfecting its harvesting in the wild, the Dutch East India Company began to grow and cultivate its own trees.

At the end of the eighteenth century, the English ousted the Dutch, but by then the monopoly of cinnamon had lessened. Development and harvesting of cinnamon trees had spread to other countries, making the spice more accessible.

QUALITIES OF CINNAMON

Currently cinnamon is grown commercially in Java, Sumatra, Brazil, the West Indies, Vietnam, Madagascar, and Egypt. The best cinnamon still comes from Sri Lanka and is known as Ceylon cinnamon, or "true cinnamon."

A fine-quality cinnamon is a light yellowish-brown color and has a fragrant smell. To cultivate it, the bark of the cinnamon tree is stripped off and dried. The thin inner bark is stripped from the woody outer bark, and the long strips dry into quills.

Cinnamon and cassia both come from the bark of a small evergreen tree, but that's where the resemblance ends. Ceylon cinnamon is less dense and has a finer texture and more aromatic smell than cassia, which is sometimes labeled as cinnamon. Cassia is reddish-brown in color and is not separated from its hard outer bark before drying so the harvested bark doesn't form perfectly rolled quills like cinnamon. The flavor is also less delicate, giving it the name "bastard cinnamon."

When ground, the difference between cassia and cinnamon is also apparent—the powder of true cinnamon is lighter in color and has a much finer texture.

The chemical composition of cassia is also very similar to that of cinnamon and contains many of the same active ingredients. Although this chapter is about the medicinal benefits of cinnamon, you should know that the United States Pharmacopeia recognizes oil of cassia as oil of cinnamon. Therefore, any cinnamon supplement you take may very well be cassia.

In the Western world, cinnamon is used in everyday products like toothpaste, detergents, soaps, lotions, massage oils, mouthwash, and other pharmaceutical products.

MEDICINAL PROPERTIES OF CINNAMON

So now we get to what cinnamon can do to improve health. In its various forms—powder, oil, incense—cinnamon has a lot to offer. Among its many uses, cinnamon is a potent antifungal and antibacterial agent, helps with type 2 diabetes, lowers cholesterol, and its very smell is considered a brain booster! A little household hint: include cinnamon in sachets to repel moths.

Cinnamon is comprised of three main elements: cinnamaldehyde, cinnamyl acetate, and cinnamyl alcohol, which are found in the essential oils from its bark. Many of cinnamon's medicinal properties come from these essential oils.

Help for Diabetics

Cinnamon's ability to reduce blood sugar in diabetics was discovered by accident. In a study that examined the effects of common foods on blood sugar, apple pie, usually spiced with cinnamon, was included. "We expected it to be bad," said Richard Anderson of the U.S. Department of Agriculture's Human Nutrition Research Center in Beltsville, Maryland. "But it helped."

Diabetes is a disease in which the body is unable to produce or properly use insulin. When food is digested by the body, it is converted into blood sugar, or glucose. As blood sugar levels rise, the pancreas releases the hormone insulin. Insulin moves glucose from the bloodstream to places where it can be used as fuel such as muscle, fat, and liver cells.

With type 2 diabetes, the pancreas is unable to produce enough insulin to control blood glucose levels. Often the body doesn't react well to insulin. High blood sugar can cause serious long-term damage to organs, including eyes, kidneys, and nerves.

Researcher Dr. Alam Kahn of the NWFP Agricultural University in Peshawar, Pakistan, conducted a study using sixty volunteers with type 2 diabetes. The subjects were given, in capsule form, 1, 3, or 6 grams of cinnamon powder per day after meals for twenty days. Within weeks, blood sugar levels averaged 20 percent lower than a control group. Interestingly enough, the group that took the smallest amount of cinnamon, 1 gram, continued with significantly improved blood sugar levels.

Not coincidentally, after the volunteers in the other two groups stopped taking cinnamon, their blood sugar levels started to escalate again.

A study published in February 2004 showed that cinnamon can prevent insulin resistance in rats that were fed a high-fructose diet. The rats, given cinnamon extract, were able to respond and utilize the sugar in their blood as well as rats fed a normal diet.

As it turns out, a chemical compound found in cinnamon mimics insulin and activates its receptor to work with and augment insulin in cells. The ingredient is a water-soluble polyphenol called MHCP.

The effects of MHCP can also benefit non-diabetics who have blood sugar problems.

Lowers Cholesterol

Results from Khan's same study also showed that volunteers' blood level of fats (triglycerides) and LDL, or "bad" cholesterol, were lowered. These levels are partially controlled by insulin.

In the forty-day tests of the study participants, all the patients had improved triglyceride levels, with between 23 and 30 percent reductions. In very encouraging results, the group that took the most cinnamon—6 grams—had the best triglyceride levels.

Blood cholesterol levels also declined by an average of 19 percent, and LDL cholesterol averaged a decline of about 17 percent. Effects on HDL, or "good" cholesterol, were minor.

Recent USDA reports show that patients who take less than a half teaspoon of cinnamon daily experienced an up to 20 percent decrease of lowered cholesterol and triglyceride levels.

Reduces High Blood Pressure

The USDA is currently conducting three ongoing studies on the effects of cinnamon in hypertension. The evidence that cinnamon is an antihypertensive is mostly anecdotal, so people are anxiously awaiting the results of those tests.

Antibacterial and Antifungal Agent

Traditionally used as a preservative for meat, cinnamon has recently been studied for its ability to stop the growth of bacteria. It has proven to be so effective that it has prevented the growth of most bacteria and fungi, including the stubborn yeast *Candida albicans.*

Studies have demonstrated that the condition of AIDS patients suffering from oral *Candida* (thrush) improves after the application of cinnamon oil. Cinnamon's antimicrobial properties also have an inhibitory effect on the bacteria that causes ulcers, *Heliobacter pylori.*

Cinnamon's ability is so powerful that it's convincing the world of modern medicine that it can be used as a food preservative alternative. In a food study, a few drops of cinnamon were added to about 3 ounces of carrot broth and then refrigerated. Without the oil, the pathogenic *Bacillus cereus* flourished in the cold temperature, where cinnamon oil prevented its growth for up to sixty days.

As a wash, it's also been used to treat fungal infections such as athlete's foot.

Relieves Intestinal Distress

Cinnamon has traditionally been used as a carminative in cases of flatulent dyspepsia, intestinal colic, diarrhea, and nausea. It's been approved by German health authorities to treat mild gastrointestinal spasms and appetite loss. The tannin components in cinnamon bark are thought to be responsible for its power as an antidiarrheal agent.

Prevents Cold/Flu

The Chinese have used cinnamon as a remedy for influenza and colds for centuries, brewing it as a tea mixed with ginger at the onset of a cold. They would swallow a small pinch of powdered cinnamon to warm cold hands and feet, especially at night.

Anticlotting

Platelets are the cells in the blood that clump together to stop bleeding at the site of trauma or physical injury. But if the platelets clot too much, they can obstruct blood flow, especially in aging patients.

Cinnamon's cinnamaldehyde has been studied for its effect on platelets and its ability to prevent unwanted clotting. Cinnamaldehyde inhibits the release of arachidonic acid—an inflammatory fatty acid in platelet membranes—making it an anti-inflammatory as well.

Boosts Brain Function

In a study that tested cognitive processing, participants were exposed to four odorant conditions: peppermint, jasmine, cinnamon, and no odor. Cinnamon surfaced as clearly the most effective in improved test scores while working on a computer-based program in the areas of attentional processes, virtual-recognition memory, working memory, and visual-motor speed.

The results of this study are inspiring researchers to study cinnamon's effect on improving cognitive capabilities in elderly patients, on patients with cognitive-decline diseases, such as Alzheimer's, and on people who suffer from test anxiety.

DOSAGE

The German *Commission E Monograph* suggests 2 to 4 grams (approximately 1/2 to 1 teaspoon) per day.

A tea can be prepared by boiling 1/2 teaspoon of cinnamon powder for ten to fifteen minutes. It can be drunk two to three times daily with meals.

Cinnamon essential oil is very powerful; only a few drops should be used for no longer than a period of several days.

Cinnamon capsules are commercially available. Potency varies, so follow the manufacturer's instructions.

Store powdered cinnamon and cinnamon sticks in airtight glass containers in a cool, dry, and dark place. Fresh cinnamon should have a sweet smell, and if that smell is missing, it's probably time to replace your cinnamon.

SIDE EFFECTS/CONTRAINDICATIONS

Cinnamon has been used as a cooking spice for thousands of years without any discernible harm or side effects. It is not a common allergen, but people with a known allergy to cinnamon or Peruvian blossom should avoid it.

Chronic use may cause sensitivity in the lining of the mouth, tongue inflammation, inflammation around the mouth; skin irritation and increased perspiration have also been reported. It can also increase intestinal activity because it may irritate the GI tract.

As a supplement, patients should use only small amounts initially.

Cinnamon is not recommended for use as a supplement by pregnant or nursing women exceeding amounts normally found in foods.

As always, patients should consult with a physician before using cinnamon as part of a daily supplement regimen.

WHY IT'S HOT!

With the incidence of obesity, diabetes, and pre-diabetic metabolic syndrome growing in the U.S. population at record rates, the old kitchen standby that your mom used in everything from apple pie to spice cake—cinnamon—is showing an amazing potential to lower blood sugar levels. A water-soluble polyphenol called MHCP is cinnamon's active agent in blood-sugar moderation, and it has the potential to significantly benefit diabetics, pre-diabetics, and non-diabetics with blood sugar problems.

In addition, researchers have demonstrated that taking less than half a teaspoon of cinnamon a day can lower blood cholesterol levels by 19 percent and LDL cholesterol by 17 percent. At the same time, cinnamon has negligible effects on HDL, or "good" cholesterol.

Cinnamon also has potent antibacterial and antifungal properties, having been used since ancient times to preserve meat. And the list goes on: cinnamon can relieve intestinal stress, prevent colds and flu, prevent clotting, and boost brain function. So while cinnamon isn't the latest, most fashionable supplement available, it may be one of the most useful in promoting health and helping to prevent a host of modern-day maladies.

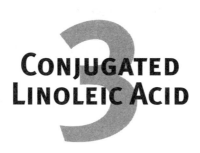

CONJUGATED
LINOLEIC ACID

L ike so many other scientific breakthroughs, CLA, or conjugated linoleic acid, was discovered accidentally. In
1978, the researcher Michael Pariza was studying the effect
of heat on burning fat to determine if the byproducts were
carcinogenic. Pariza identified substances that demonstrated antimutagenic properties and began work on isolating
these particular chemicals and found a new nutrient he
called conjugated linoleic acid. His studies found that:

- CLA has powerful anticancer potential.
- It helps prevent the clogging of arteries.
- It helps the body deal with the cascade of effects
  that occurs when an infection sets in, helping animals, and, potentially, humans.
- It can help cut body fat while building lean muscle
  tissue, which can create healthier, leaner animals.
- Though this question is debated, many researchers
  believe that CLA is a powerful antioxidant.

Dr. Pariza observed that the amount of CLA in today's typical diet is much lower than it used to be—and much lower than it should be.

By definition, CLA is part of a group of acids called essential fatty acids, which are beneficial to the body. The body produces all the fatty acids it needs except three— linoleic acid, arachidonic acid, and linolenic acid. Much the way certain vitamins like vitamin C are essential to good health and are not produced naturally, these acids are essential, hence their name—essential fatty acids. The body can produce linolenic acid and arachidonic acid from linoleic acid, so in one sense, the only vital fatty acid is linoleic acid.

Linoleic acid can be viewed as a highway of some fifty-eight atoms of carbon, oxygen, and hydrogen. Carbon is the center line, with the hydrogen and oxygen acting as the cars traveling along the way. (Thousands of chemicals contain these three elements in nature. It is the order of these cars, and the varied shapes of the highway, that lead to many different kinds of chemicals.)

The highway of linoleic acid is curved like a mountain switchback. Conjugated linoleic acid is basically a straighter version of linoleic acid. Scientists have studied CLA at least since the 1930s. These studies show that bacteria in the stomach convert linoleic acid into CLA.

CLA occurs naturally in many foods, including some vegetable oils, which are the best sources for linoleic acid, but the best source of CLA is beef, veal, and certain dairy products. Dr. Mark Cook, who began working with Dr. Pariza around 1990, said the reason that sheep and cows and similar animals provide higher sources of CLA is because these animals are ruminants—they have multiple stomachs that allow bacteria to produce linoleic acid.

There are several forms of CLA, depending on the atomic chain of chemical bonds. They vary based on where the double bond of carbon atoms occurs. Which ones are most effective in providing nutrition, or if they are equally effective, is still a question that's unresolved.

What has been resolved is that CLA is one of the most important, and most exciting, nutrients isolated in recent years. And there's good reason to look at supplementing it into your diet. Why? Because we may not be getting as much of it as we once did, particularly in the United States.

Cattle and other animals have traditionally eaten fresh grasses as a way of getting nutrition, but agricultural development makes it more efficient and cost-effective to provide cattle feed grains and other means of nutrition, instead of natural grasses. This means that cattle today provide much less CLA in their beef than those of only a generation ago. One study conducted in Australia showed that cattle there had more than twice the amount of CLA than their American counterparts. The reason may well be differences in feeding patterns.

CLA AS AN ANTIOXIDANT

The importance of antioxidants such as vitamin C, selenium, and vitamin E is common knowledge today. But what many people don't realize is that nature provides many different antioxidants, such as proanthocyanidins (often known as pycnogenol), quercetin (common in many fruits), and selenium (a mineral).

CLA may be another antioxidant emerging from the research. Dr. Pariza and others found in a 1991 experiment that in the test tube, CLA was effective in battling free radicals. It helped prevent damage to the DNA inside the cells. Dr. Pariza reports in another paper that, "Our hypothesis is that the antioxidant activity of CLA may at least in part explain its anti-carcinogenic effect." That would mean that one way CLA prevents cancer is because it blocks these dangerous free radicals. (Other theories about how it fights cancer include breaking down the chemicals that cause cancer into others that don't. All the theories may be true in specific situations, and none may be.)

But like many other emerging, exciting areas of scientific inquiry, this idea that CLA is an antioxidant has its doubters. Researchers J. J. van den Berg, N. E. Cook, and D. L. Tribble wanted to see if CLA protected fatty membranes comprised of a substance called palmitoyl-2-linoleoyl phosphatidylcholine (PLPC) from the damage of biologic oxidation. In research published in 1995, scientists compared CLA's effect to the well-known antioxidant vitamin E. While vitamin E protected well, CLA did relatively little. They also found that CLA did not become a mineral chelator, an agent that helps natural minerals become available biologically. They bluntly said, "On the basis of our observations, a role for CLA as an antioxidant does not seem plausible."

Another study in 1995, however, showed that CLA can break down into other substances, called feran derivatives, that do act as antioxidants. As in all emerging sciences, debates ensue among honest, dedicated researchers. CLA may not, in and of itself, be an antioxidant. Perhaps it acts as an antioxidant under only certain circumstances. Perhaps components of CLA act like antioxidants. That is the state of the research today. (Indeed, Dr. Pariza says such debates are common in the field of antioxidants.)

CLA AND CANCER

What is important to remember is that in numerous animal models, CLA protected against the dangers of many different kinds of cancer in animals, and that, according to scientists, it is one of the most potent cancer-preventing substances of its kind known to science. Whether the cause of this effect was because of CLA or because of some other reason really isn't that important.

No one is asserting that CLA is a cancer drug. But it may be something that would be useful in addition to other cancer treatments. It is something to consider to lower your risks and, perhaps, lessen the effects of treatment. It should not be considered a treatment option on its own.

In fact, some of the earliest studies done on CLA were to see if it could block the development of cancer. Dr. Pariza and his colleagues at the University of Wisconsin–Madison's Food Research Institute took extracts from beef that they knew had "mutagen modulators" (this was before they isolated CLA). They took two groups of mice; to one group they applied the extract to their skin. To the other group, they did not apply the extract on the skin. Then, in both groups, researchers applied a cancer-causing substance called dimethylbenzanthracene—DMBA—to the skin.

Sixteen weeks later, researchers counted the mice that had tumors and how many tumors each of those mice had. The number of mice with tumors was 20 percent lower when given the beef extract, and, significantly, the numbers of tumors on the mice that did develop cancer was half what it was on the untreated mice. This meant that this extract could, perhaps, prevent some cancers in mice and slow tumors after they develop. (Today, Pariza writes that CLA inhibits cancer development at various stages, from initiation to metastasis.) After isolating CLA, Pariza and others found that it also cut the incidence of skin tumors.

Scientist Clement Ip at the Roswell Park Cancer Institute in Buffalo, N.Y., conducted a similar study using DMBA with rats, this time feeding different amounts of CLA into the diet over a longer period of time. Ip and his team measured how many breast tumors these rats developed. As might have been expected from the earlier research, 20 percent fewer animals developed the tumors—among those receiving the most CLA—than the rats that received none, and the total number of tumors that developed was 60 percent less. In general, the data demonstrated that the more CLA, the greater the protective effect.

This is significant to humans because many researchers see a link between a woman's consumption of fat and her risk of getting breast cancer, and CLA could help modulate that risk. Any research that will discover new ways to reduce the incidence of breast cancer is useful. Today in the United States, as many as one in eight women will contract the dreaded disease.

In 1990, Dr. Pariza and his colleagues also found a lower incidence of cancers in parts of the stomach. Rats were administered 2-amino-3-methylimidazo [4,5-f] quinoline, which can give them colon cancer. Again, the total number of aberrant growths was lower for those given CLA compared with those given safflower oil, which is rich in essential oils but not so high in CLA.

Does this mean that CLA will prevent cancer in humans? Perhaps. You might even say probably—in some circumstances. Still, science can be imprecise in predicting cancers from animal models to humans, and scientific tests must be controlled in ways that don't mimic the complexities and confounding factors of daily life. Few of us, for example, will be exposed daily to DMBA. Therefore, all the science says for certain is that CLA seems to hinder the development of cancer in these animals when the cancer is caused by one particular substance. That's a little way, at least, from saying it prevents cancers in humans.

But the animal models are encouraging and statistically significant. In fact, some scientists maintain without hedging that CLA has an anticarcinogenic effect. Ip himself says, "CLA is more powerful than any other fatty acid in modulating tumor development." Indeed, so excited have many scientists become that some say one day governments may want to fortify our foods with CLA much the way we fortify our morning bran flakes with vitamin C. Furthermore, since at least several ways of giving different species of animals cancer have been studied, and in all of the tests, cancer was hindered, it gives better evidence to the notion that CLA hinders cancer in humans as well. Pariza wrote, "Few anti-carcinogens, and certainly no other known fatty acids, are as effective as CLA in inhibiting carcinogenesis in these models." This is clear language from a scientist who believes this to be a powerful nutrient in the war against cancer. But until more human research is completed, any claims that CLA prevents cancer in humans is still preliminary.

Additionally, since the breakdown and transformation of fats and fatty acids like CLA occur in the liver, CLA may have unknown effects on this vital organ. One study showed that fats increase in the liver with an increase of CLA in the diet. Could this lead to an increased risk of liver cancer? Scientists do not have a complete answer to that question either. Dr. Pariza says, however, that such problems of fat accumulation do not occur in higher mammals and are specific to mice and some rats.

CLA and Atherosclerosis

CLA may well have benefits in the battle against heart disease as well. The leading cause of death in the United States is heart disease or related diseases of the circulatory system. Indeed, U.S. statistics show that about half the people in the United States succumb to heart and related circulatory diseases.

Modern medicine has made great progress in battling these conditions, and researchers have discovered that a healthy lifestyle can help the heart. Indeed, as almost everyone knows, balanced nutrition, lower stress, and plenty of exercise can create greater health and lower the risk of heart attacks and other heart conditions.

CLA also seems to possess the ability to cut the risk of arterial disease. Pariza and two colleagues, Kisun Lee and David Kritchevsky, studied a group of twelve rabbits that were fed a diet high in fat and cholesterol. They gave six of the rabbits CLA. In the academic journal *Atherosclerosis,* researchers reported that two dangerous compounds, LDL cholesterol and triglycerides, were "markedly lower" in the six rabbits that consumed diets supplemented with CLA.

When the scientists examined the rabbits' aortas—the largest artery leading from the heart—they also found significantly less blockage than in the rabbits that didn't have CLA supplementation. They noted that, "CLA appears to be hypocholesterolemic and anti-atherogenic." This is pretty bold stuff for cautious scientists. Though the words are complex, the statement is clear: CLA seems to cut cholesterol and help prevent vein-clogging plaque buildup.

This finding surprised Dr. Pariza. Science has demonstrated that straightened fatty acids (trans-fatty acids) of which CLA is one, usually tend to increase the risk of heart disease. Pariza said it only made sense to test CLA with this kind of science. Indeed, the best he would hope for would be no effect. In 1996, another group of scientists studied atherosclerosis in hamsters by supplementing diets with CLA. The CLA didn't cut the amount of cholesterol in the blood within three months, but it did cut the amount of fatty buildup in the hamsters' aortas.

What's the bottom line on heart disease and CLA? Because two different types of animals show less clogging of the arteries, it seems clear that a good chance exists for the same thing to happen in humans. As with the cancer research, solid studies in humans need to be conducted before researchers can definitely say that CLA can cut your risk of heart disease.

But until that time, the news is good: A nutritional regimen that includes solid antioxidants like vitamin C and vitamin A, that includes magnesium, coenzyme Q10, and that includes other important circulatory system fortifiers would likely benefit from CLA. Couple that nutrition with a healthy lifestyle, and your chances of living longer and living better will likely increase.

CLA AND THE CATABOLIC CASCADE

The next time you are immunized (a flu shot, etc.), notice how run-down you feel for a day or so afterwards. It's as if you have a small dose of the disease.

In some respects you do. In reality, however, that malaise comes from your body's own response to an invasion. When the immune system goes on the offensive, it puts out hormones called cytokines. Those cytokines cause fever and pain.

Doctors call this process the catabolic cascade. It is our body that produces it. Cytokines are involved in more than just stimulating the immune system—they also determine how the body accumulates fat, how arteries and veins accumulate deposits, and how the body sometimes experiences rapid weight loss during an illness. CLA changes how cytokines work, but how it does so is not fully understood.

During an illness, not only does the immune system kick into action, but tissue growth also slows. As a result, muscle mass can be lost, not just because of a loss of appetite, but also because of the degradation of muscle tissue. For a poultry farmer, for example, this can be significant. As young chicks come into contact with bacteria, their immune systems fire up, activating cytokines that can stunt growth and shrink the farmer's profits.

Dr. Mark Cook was working on this problem in 1990 at the University of Wisconsin–Madison and in collaboration with Dr. Pariza wanted to determine if CLA had an effect on this problem.

During the study, rat pups were injected with endotoxin, the substances that bacteria produce to do their damage. This injection activated their immune systems. They also did the same thing in two studies using chicks. In all three studies, the weight loss was about half of what it was during the other studies.

In a study published in 1994, researchers also injected endotoxin into mice. To some, they gave CLA, to others they didn't. After three days, the scientists weighed the mice and discovered that those who also received CLA in their diets lost much less weight. Indeed, after three days they weighed as much as the control group, which received no endotoxin at all. The CLA-fed group also had a much better appetite than those that received no CLA with endotoxin. They also had a higher muscle mass.

That last finding was significant. Other studies have shown that CLA also cuts the amount of food converted to fat. In an era of increasing battles with the bulge, CLA seems to show great promise. (The involvement of weight gain with the immune system and cytokines indicates that working with cytokines may be how CLA affects body fat accumulation.)

This research raised some new questions: While CLA can help cut the effects of immune stimulation, does it do that at the expense of making our immune systems less effective? Does CLA affect how the body battles disease? The answers? The 1993 studies measured several immune functions, and, if anything, determined that the immune system worked better with CLA supplementation.

Again, these are animal—not human—studies. However, they do involve more than one kind of animal, suggesting its usefulness to humans.

Let's speculate for a minute. When CLA cuts the catabolic cascade, doesn't it make sense that the body would feel better, if only because the appetite is better? When CLA cuts weight loss, couldn't that have immense benefits for patients suffering from long-term illnesses—including those illnesses that affect the immune system—who grow weak from a loss of muscle tone and weight?

For the animal industry, of course, this nutrient clearly means better production methods and healthier animals. For those same animals, it seems possible to speculate that CLA may actually work as a growth factor for their young.

For humans, this nutrient could mean feeling better and stronger while the body fights off disease.

This research has one other interesting side effect. Cook says that during much of the research, graduate students helping in the work would continually report that animals were eating less. Indeed, the animals ate up to 30 percent less while gaining weight or helping the immune system.

If all animals in the world were fed CLA, and it cut feed intake by 30 percent, this would have strong implications on world starvation and feed efficiency.

CLA AND BODY FAT

Of all the health concerns facing Americans today, few are as important and daunting as weight loss and body fat. In a recent decade, Americans gained an average of 8 pounds each. That's on the order of one million tons of flab—two billion total American pounds. So large is the current girth that as many as two in three Americans could be termed overweight. Being overweight and having excess fat increases the risk of heart disease, some forms of cancer, and diabetes. That collection of health challenges would be difficult enough, but being overweight creates many other problems, including battles with self-esteem.

History and culture have conditioned us to believe that being overweight means lacking self-control and being gluttons, when in reality these beliefs aren't true. So many more factors are involved. Each person has a different metabolism. Certain nutrients can meet different needs, and a lack of those nutrients can lead to fat retention.

CLA may be one of those nutrients, one of those factors in our diets that can change our shapes and that have nothing to do with self-control, just nutritional luck and knowledge.

In a study of rats, twenty-eight days after beginning the study, body fat in those that ate CLA was 58 percent less than in those that didn't consume any (10.13 percent body fat versus 4.34 percent body fat, a highly significant difference). Also, the percent of muscle was about 1 percent greater in animals that consumed CLA. The weights of both sets of animals were about the same. (Muscle weighs more than fat. This can mean that you won't necessarily lose weight with CLA, but would gain muscle mass, which is tighter and more shapely.)

The research in this area is slightly newer, but it has been reproduced in studies on other animals. Since more than one kind of animal has demonstrated that body fat is lower with CLA supplementation, it will be likely to benefit humans as well.

In July 1997, preliminary results of one of the first human studies involving CLA showed promising preliminary results. For three months in 1997, twenty volunteers participated in a study, daily consuming an amount of slightly more than 1 gram of CLA at breakfast, lunch, and dinner. Three months later, their weights and body-fat percentages were measured. Half of the group took a placebo. The average weight of the ten who took CLA dropped by about 5 pounds (not enough to be statistically significant), but the body fat percentage dropped by about 15 to 20 percent, or from 21.3 percent of average body fat to 17 percent of body fat. Meanwhile, the group taking a placebo had little or no effect on either.

Half of the people in the study were men and half were women. Two people in the study dropped out because they experienced unpleasant gastrointestinal symptoms. One of those who dropped out was in the placebo group, the other was in the group taking CLA.

Nobody would suggest that CLA supplementation would be a pill freeing you to sit slug-like on the couch to watch *Seinfeld* reruns. A healthy, weight-conscious lifestyle requires many factors including exercise. As far as science can tell, CLA may not be essential the way certain vitamins are. If you consume no vitamin C, you can expect to get scurvy and die. There are no known deficiency diseases associated with an absence of CLA. The Japanese, for example, get very little CLA in their diets, but they also eat food very low in fat, and their lives are among the longest in the world. So, the role of CLA supplementation in regulating weight is most useful for those with a typically high-fat Western diet. As the science grows, it seems clear that CLA will lead to better health and more hope for people struggling with excess body fat.

How Much CLA Is the Right Amount?

That is one question for researchers to answer with detailed human studies, but if you extrapolate from university studies on animals, it could be between 2 and 6 grams a day. (Some animal studies were actually at higher levels, to 0.5 percent in weight of a day's calories.)

Some Final Thoughts on CLA

Watch the labels closely on supplements advertising that they contain CLA. CLA is present in many foods (two of the best natural sources of CLA are beef and veal) and some marketers have capitalized on CLA science by simply putting vegetable oil in their supplements. Only a few supplements provide high levels of CLA. Select only those products that do.

CLA is not like aspirin, in that it takes a few weeks, perhaps three, for its effects to be noticeable.

To get enough CLA from hamburgers, you would probably have to eat about 2 pounds a day, not something that's recommended given beef's high fat content.

In general, plants have virtually no CLA.

Aside from questions about liver cancer, no adverse side effects have been reported in the scientific literature concerning CLA. CLA can probably be taken safely with other nutritional supplements, but fat-absorbing supplements like chitosan may actually absorb CLA, so it's best to avoid taking the two products at the same time. Consider taking CLA in the morning and chitosan after high-fat meals.

Why It's Hot!

Important research results are now emerging. According to Cook, in animal studies that monitored quantities of fat and muscle, researchers noticed that overall weight was consistently up. Most recently, as-yet-unpublished results show that bone mass increased in pigs that consumed

CLA. This has huge implications for research into osteo-porosis, and research in this area is under way.

Scores of scientists in the United States are now study-ing CLA. The results of their research from human studies and other long-term clinical trials will give broad indica-tions of the use of this previously unrecognized natural nutrient.

Why would CLA be involved in so many functions? If human studies hold true, and the expectation is that they will, you might consider CLA to be the next aspirin or the next vitamin C. Vital, remarkable nutrients seem to work on a basic level and affect a variety of body systems. This is the case with CLA.

What remarkable science that's emerged from a char-coal grill!

CRANBERRY

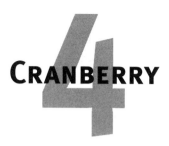

Although a member of the berry family, cranberries (*Vaccinium macrocarpon*) don't enjoy quite the same fame as other sweet summer varieties. But what cranberries lack in popularity, they make up for in potency. Science shows that the tart, red berries are the most beneficial to your health of any berry species—better than any other common fruits for antioxidant activity. With the incidence of cancer, heart disease, and other chronic conditions rising throughout the world, research on cranberries has increased to understand and utilize the immense possibilities of these healthy berries.

CRANBERRY COUNTRY

Would you be surprised to learn that the tradition of cranberry sauce on the Thanksgiving table is as old as the holiday itself? Cranberries are indigenous to America, and have grown abundantly in the wild for centuries. Native Americans along the East Coast enjoyed the wild berries cooked with maple syrup or honey, and most likely shared their favorite treat with colonists at early Thanksgiving feasts. Native Americans made use of cranberries for other reasons too, most commonly to make red dye and to clean wounds. By the beginning of the eighteenth century, the colonists had begun exporting cranberries back to England.

Cranberries continue to be primarily cultivated in North America, thanks in part to a discovery by Henry Hall at his farm in Dennis, Massachusetts, in 1840. Hall observed that the berries flourished when sand was fortuitously swept into his bog by strong winds, because the sand stifled the growth of shallow weeds while supporting the deep-rooted cranberry bushes. The United States produces 154,000 tons of cranberries each year, the majority of which come from Wisconsin and Massachusetts.

CRANBERRIES AND URINARY HEALTH: THE RESEARCH

Recent studies suggest that cranberries and cranberry juice may help maintain a healthy urinary tract by preventing urinary tract infections. Some researchers are at odds with one another about why this is the case, however. One theory is that the hippuric acid present in cranberries is responsible. Early studies on cranberry proposed that the hippuric acid helps acidify urine enough to prevent harmful bacteria from developing into an infection. However, several similar studies have failed to prove this theory or demonstrate that hippuric acid can reach bacteriostatic levels within the urinary tract.

More recent research has proposed a different reason for cranberries' urinary health benefits. Scientists have turned their attention to the cranberry's ability to prevent harmful bacteria from adhering to the urinary tract altogether. A 1998 study suggests that certain compounds called proanthocyanidins found in cranberries function similarly to the body's Tamm-Horsfall glycoprotein, which keeps bacteria from adhering to bladder cells. Urinary tract infections (UTIs) are caused by a class of bacteria known as *fimbriated gram negative rods*, which includes the *E. coli*, *Porteus*, and *Pseudomona* species. The fimbriae of these pathogens—the fringe-like material surrounding the bacteria—allows it to attach itself to the epithelial cells of the urinary tract and create an infection. However, an in vitro study published in 1988 showed that bacterial fimbriae are less likely to stick to the urinary tract when cranberry juice, or the urine of someone who drank cranberry juice, is present. The results also suggested that cranberry is more effective as a preventive measure than as a cure for existing infections.

A large double-blind, placebo-controlled trial conducted in 1994 stands out as one of the more effective human trials measuring cranberry's effect on urinary health. Researchers arranged for 153 elderly women from a nursing home to drink 300 ml (10 ounces) of cranberry juice per day. The results confirmed a trend towards fewer UTIs in the juice-drinking participants, and showed that only 15 percent of the group was found to have bacteria in their urine, compared to 28 percent of the placebo group.

Another notable cranberry/urinary health study tested the benefits of cranberry supplements. Ten women aged twenty-eight to forty-four participated in the double-blind crossover placebo-controlled trial for six months. By the end of the study, twenty-one UTIs had occurred: fifteen during the placebo stage of the trial versus only six during the treatment stage.

In addition to the UTI-preventing benefits, cranberry may also have other positive effects on the urinary system. A few preliminary uncontrolled studies have shown that cranberry juice may help reduce the odor of urine, as well as the occasional burning sensation that accompanies urination. Further research is still necessary to confirm these benefits.

POWERFUL PROANTHOCYANIDINS

The latest research points to cranberry's exceptional concentration of bioflavonoids to explain its many health benefits. Science uses the umbrella term *bioflavonoids* for the many healthful phytochemicals found in fruits and vegetables, herbs, grains, legumes, and nuts. Bioflavonoids frequently have antioxidant properties—some have been found to possess antiviral, anti-inflammatory, and antihistamine abilities as well. Proanthocyanidins are just one of the many types of bioflavonoids that cranberries contain, but research suggests it is one of the most beneficial.

Proanthocyanidins are potent antioxidants that are most abundantly found in blue, red, or purple fruits—cranberry being one of the most plentiful sources. In addition to their great antioxidant properties, certain proanthocyanidins like proanthocyanidin A-1 have additional advantages for the body, including the anti-adherence property studied in connection with urinary health and a host of other conditions.

MORE ANTI-ADHERENCE ABILITIES

Fighting urinary tract infections is just the beginning of cranberry's anti-adherence abilities. A number of other diseases and conditions may also be mitigated by cranberry's powerful proanthocyanidins.

Ulcers

A recent discovery suggests that most gastric ulcers form because of harmful *Heliobacter pylori* bacteria that adhere to the lining of the stomach wall. Results from a 2002 in vitro study published in *Critical Reviews in Food Science and Nutrition* indicate that cranberry juice may help prevent *H. pylori* from adhering to the stomach lining. In this respect, ulcer sufferers may benefit from cranberries in much the same way as those with urinary tract infections.

Oral Health

A different study in 2002 discussed cranberry's possible anti-adherence effects on oral disease. The study noted that a mouthwash containing a unique cranberry compound was able to break up the dental plaque formed by a number of oral bacteria and decrease the salivary level of the *Streptococcus mutans* that causes tooth decay.

Genital Herpes

The most controversial research on cranberry's anti-adherence abilities involves studies on the genital herpes virus. Laboratory work published in the October 2004 issue of the *Journal of Science, Food and Agriculture* shows that the proanthocyanidin A-1 phytonutrients found in cranberry may in fact be effective in preventing the attachment and penetration of the herpes simplex virus. But like cranberries' effects on the urinary tract, the benefits are only preventative.

FIGHTING FREE RADICALS

Recent studies have shown that air pollution, cigarette smoke, pesticides, contaminated water, and even the food we eat can produce free radicals. Free radicals are unstable oxygen molecules that cause damage to other healthy cells, often referred to as oxidation damage. This damage can impair the proper functioning of the immune system, which then can lead to infections, chronic disease, and cancer. Cranberries are a rich source of antioxidants that can help kill harmful free radicals and protect cellular DNA from both oxidative damage and cell mutations that can lead to cancer.

Cancerous tumors grow out of abnormal, uncontrolled cell division instigated by free radicals. Science tells us that a healthy diet of antioxidants, like those contained in cranberries, may have the ability to stop tumors before they start. In a 2002 study, several cranberry compounds—particularly proanthocyanidins—demonstrated a toxicity to various cancer tumor cells, including breast, prostate, lung, cervical, and leukemia cancer cells. This study, as well as several contemporary studies, also found that whole cranberries, as opposed to cranberry juice, are the most effective in fighting cancer cells. Researchers have concluded that the active compounds in whole cranberries help prevent cancer and decrease the growth of tumors by halting cell cycle progression and causing cells to suffer programmed cell death.

Looking for an antiaging miracle? Antioxidants may be a start. As people age, free radicals can wreak havoc throughout the body, accelerating the aging process, and causing losses in eyesight and motor and cognitive function. Proanthocyanidins found in cranberries work to combat many of the effects we see as a normal part of the aging process. They accomplish this partly through their ability to enhance immune resistance. Proanthocyanidins make up one of the most important immune system nutrients to come along in the past fifty years. Because they remain in the body for three full days and are also bioavailable, they can be distributed to virtually every organ and tissue. A healthy immune system is vital to slowing the aging process for a long and healthy life.

The proanthocyanidins found in cranberries work to increase peripheral circulation, and thus may help improve vision. They help prevent free radical damage and reinforce the collagen structures in the retina. In clinical trials of patients with various types of retinal disease, including macular degeneration, all patients given proanthocyanidins showed significant improvement following therapy. Health professionals monitoring the effect of proanthocyanidins have reported that they have also helped in the prevention and treatment of glaucoma.

Proanthocyanidins are one of only a few antioxidant sources that cross the blood/brain barrier to protect neural tissue. This property may explain why proanthocyanidins have been able to help patients with such nerve diseases as multiple sclerosis (MS). Other diseases associated with aging may also be helped by proanthocyanidins. Preliminary animal studies on rats have produced compelling evidence that cranberry antioxidants can help keep the mind sharp and free from other neurological damage by fighting free radicals in the brain as well as the body.

LIFE AT THE TOP

When it comes to antioxidant power, cranberries enjoy a view from the top. According to several topical studies done by universities throughout the country, cranberries contain more antioxidants than any other common fruit and subsequently, the greatest potential to fight free radicals and harmful oxidation.

The University of Scranton, University of Massachusetts–Dartmouth, and Cornell University recently conducted studies in which they compared cranberries with a variety of other fruits and fruit juices. Each of the three studies concluded that cranberry ranks number one in antioxidant phenols among common fruits and fruit juices, and that the phytochemical powerhouse may even outpower certain healthy vegetables like broccoli by as much as five to one.

THE HEARTENING EFFECTS OF CRANBERRY

The battle against heart disease has a new weapon. Just as science begins to delve into the causes and factors involved with the nation's number-one killer, timely new research shows that cranberry's antioxidant power may help reduce cholesterol levels and protect against heart disease.

One in vitro study from the University of Scranton suggests that the same cranberry antioxidants that protect against cancer and other chronic diseases may help protect LDL cholesterol from oxidation—a condition that recent experimental studies have discovered is a key factor leading to hardening of the arteries and heart disease. Similar animal studies have concluded that cranberries may also help decrease total cholesterol and LDL cholesterol levels.

Further investigation suggests that one particular cranberry antioxidant, pterostilbene, may hold the key to cranberries' "heartening" effects. A study completed by the USDA Agricultural Research Service compared pterostilbene's cholesterol-lowering ability with that of a ciprofibrate, a common lipid-lowering drug. The results of the study concluded that pterostilbene was more likely to stimulate cholesterol metabolism than ciprofibrate, and therefore, keep cholesterol levels at healthy, balanced levels.

Cranberries may also play a part in maintaining blood vessel health, particularly in those with atherosclerosis. Proanthocyanidins found in cranberries help enhance capillary strength and vascular function, which helps the heart and also decreases bruising edema from injury or trauma, varicose veins, leg swelling, and retinopathy. One 2005 animal study from the University of Wisconsin–Madison revealed that a daily dose of cranberry powder for pigs with atherosclerosis increased vascular relaxation and helped their blood vessels function more like those of normal pigs. Since unhealthy blood vessels can contribute to heart disease, science continues to look at how cranberries can help prevent atherosclerotic patients from experiencing heart attacks or strokes.

A Better, Bitter Berry

The incidence of kidney stones in American adults has inexplicably risen sharply over the past few decades—primarily in white middle-aged men, but also in women and younger people as well. While doctors can't definitively explain what causes kidney, they hypothesize that genetics, other urinary or kidney infections, and even certain foods can cause stones to develop.

Kidney stones are hard stone-like masses that form when crystallized substances in urine—usually calcium, phosphate, or other mineral ions—build up on the inner walls of the kidney and ureters connecting the kidney to the bladder. Urine typically contains chemicals that prevent the crystal-like substances from forming, but these chemicals aren't present or aren't effective in some people. Luckily, cranberries may provide a viable substitute for these defective chemicals.

Cranberries contain a chemical known as quinic acid, which is unique in that it isn't broken down as it passes through the body, but instead is excreted mostly unaffected in urine. The presence of quinic acid in urine may help prevent kidney stones from forming. Clinical studies have shown that quinic acid can make urine just acidic enough to prevent calcium and phosphate ions from combining to form kidney stones, and can also reduce the amount of ionized calcium in urine by over 50 percent—a significant amount considering that 75–85 percent of kidney stones are composed of calcium salts. Some studies have also suggested that the acidity of cranberries plays a minor role in helping to clear up urinary tract infections.

SAFETY ISSUES

Cranberries contain a considerable amount of oxalates—naturally occurring substances that are found in most living things. However, when body fluids become too concentrated with oxalates they can interfere with the absorption of calcium from the body, and may aggravate existing health conditions such as kidney or gallbladder problems.

Special Instructions

Individuals taking the drug warfarin are advised to avoid cranberries, based on recent reports from the United

Kingdom that they may inhibit blood clotting activity. Persons undergoing anticancer chemotherapy and radiation should also abstain from cranberries and other supplemental antioxidants during treatment, as the antioxidants may decrease the effectiveness of the medicine.

Why It's Hot!

The recent discovery of cranberry's anti-adherence abilities on urinary tract infections has spurred further study into other potential benefits they may hold for the prevention of ulcers, oral disease, and possibly even genital herpes. Cranberries continue to reign as the most antioxidant-rich common fruit, the power of which holds great promise for the fight against cancer, aging, and macular degeneration. Cranberries' many antioxidants also play a role in helping to maintain a healthy cardiovascular system and prevent the onset of heart disease. In addition, the phytochemicals contained in cranberries, such as quinic acid, may help put off the pain and nuisance of kidney stones and help maintain a healthy urinary system.

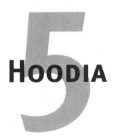

HOODIA

Long ago, the Bushmen of Africa's Kalahari desert discovered parts of a particular plant—the *Hoodia gordonii*—that can yield not only a lifesaving liquid, but also some truly amazing benefits. For centuries now, they have eaten bite-size chunks to ward off thirst and curb their appetites and eliminate hunger during long hunting trips in the wilderness.

Not only is there no running water in the Kalahari, there is virtually no surface water for most of the year. Only during the brief rainy season do the Bushmen—the most ancient group of nomadic hunter-gatherers on earth—have the luxury of a water supply. To survive during the rest of the year, they must rely on the water content of their food, the morning dew they collect from leaves, and the moisture they extract from other sources, such as underground tubers.

Besides thirst, the Bushmen, known as the San, also learned how to suppress their appetite, an important survival skill in a region where just finding enough food to eat is a never-ending challenge, especially while on a lengthy hunt, when they walk or run as much as a hundred miles in pursuit of elusive prey. To escape their distress from unending hunger pangs they'd chew on *Hoodia gordonii*.

In an interview with ABC News in 2003, Andries Steenkamp, a spokesman for the San people, said, "I learned how to eat it from my forefathers. It is my food, my water, and also a medicine for me. We San use the plant during hunting to fight off the pain of hunger and thirst."

Although it looks like a small cactus, *Hoodia gordonii*—commonly known simply as hoodia—is actually a type of milkweed. It thrives in very high temperatures, and takes years to mature.

Being a succulent, hoodia contains a lot of moisture. Although bitter tasting, it is a welcome relief when you have few, if any, alternatives for liquid sustenance in the desert. Sucking on the pulpy flesh, the Bushmen could not only quell their thirst but also ward off their hunger. In addition, according to Bushman lore, hoodia gives them enough energy to walk all day or to make love all night, and it cures a hangover and settles an upset stomach.

HOODIA COMES WEST

The first supplements containing the hoodia compound were introduced in the United States early in 2004 to aid in obesity and weight loss by suppressing appetite. Obesity doesn't just make it hard to fit into your clothes. Obesity can significantly increase your risk of chronic diseases and conditions, including

- Hypertension
- High serum cholesterol
- Type 2 diabetes
- Coronary heart disease
- Stroke
- Gallbladder disease
- Osteoarthritis
- Sleep apnea
- Respiratory problems
- Endometrial, breast, prostate, and colon cancers

WHAT IS HOODIA?

Hoodia gordonii is a succulent plant belonging to the milkweed (*Asclepiadaceae*) family that consists of approximately twenty species. Known locally as xhoba, hoodia is a leafless, spiny plant—not truly a cactus—with fleshy finger-like stems. There are rows of thorns along the stems, and the plants bear flesh-colored flowers. The flowers emit a strong smell of decaying meat, which attracts flies that lay their eggs inside and pollinate them.

Sometimes the word is spelled *hootia*, *hodia*, *hoodie*, and *hudia*. Recently, hoodia garnered a great deal of attention after being featured on CBS's *60 Minutes* and on the BBC in the United Kingdom.

The hoodia species grows in summer rainfall areas in Angola, Botswana, Namibia, and South Africa, as well as winter rainfall areas in Namibia. Only one species is found east of 26 degrees longitude, *H. currorii subsp. Lugardii*, which appears in Botswana and the Limpopo province of South Africa. Although the genus *Hoodia* is widespread in southern Africa, *Hoodia gordonii* only occurs in South Africa and Namibia despite some claims to the contrary. *Hoodia gordonii* is the only species that contains the compound that suppresses appetite. From here on out in this chapter, "hoodia" will mean *Hoodia gordonii.*

Since hoodia has been used for thousands of years by San Bushmen who needed to remain active to survive, they had little need to diet, but learned that this plant provided stamina and curbed hunger during prolonged periods without food. Besides the benefit of reducing or eliminating the desire for food, many believe hoodia also increases energy and can have an aphrodisiac-like effect on the user.

Hoodia's appetite-suppressing ingredient is a molecule similar to glucose, only stronger. The Council for Scientific and Industrial Research (CSIR) in South Africa isolated an active compound for appetite suppression from *Hoodia gordonii*, known as P57, which seems to send a signal to the hypothalamus of the brain and "tricks" the body into believing that it's no longer hungry. The result is a complete lack of appetite.

Among the many chemical compounds found in the sap of *Hoodia gordonii*, scientists in South Africa have discovered an appetite-suppressing compound with a long and complicated name they've dubbed P57. P57 is a steroidal glycoside, a steroid molecule chemically bonded to a chain of three sugar molecules.

Some years back, scientists at Brown University Medical School in Providence, Rhode Island, became interested in P57 as a means for investigating how the sense of satiety, or fullness, is induced in our brains, telling us to stop eating. Because P57 is an anorectic (an agent that suppresses appetite), they believed pinpointing the mechanism by which it acts on the brain should shed some light on this question. They found the appetite-suppressing and mood-enhancing property (ten thousand times as active as glucose) goes to the mid-brain, causing neuron nerve cells to fire as if you were full, even when you're not.

How Does It Work?

The hypothalamus is the region of the brain that contains several important centers that control body temperature, thirst, hunger, water balance, and sexual function. The hypothalamus is also closely connected with emotional activity and sleep, and functions as a center for the integration of hormonal and autonomic nervous activity through its control of pituitary secretions. The hypothalamus links the nervous system to the endocrine system.

In our bodies, the pituitary gland is often portrayed as the "master gland," since the anterior and posterior pituitary secrete a battery of hormones that collectively influence all cells and affect virtually all physiological processes. But the power behind the pituitary gland is the hypothalamus, because neurosecretory neurons within the hypothalamus secrete hormones that strictly control the secretion of hormones from the anterior pituitary. The hypothalamic hormones are referred to as releasing hormones and inhibiting hormones, reflecting their influence on anterior pituitary hormones.

Hypothalamic releasing and inhibiting hormones are carried directly to the anterior pituitary gland via hypothalamic-hypophyseal portal veins. Here, hypothalamic hormones bind to receptors on anterior pituitary cells, modulating the release of the hormone they produce.

The P57 compound found in hoodia appears to work by increasing the content of adenosine triphosphate (ATP) in nerve cells in the hypothalamus, the brain's control center for regulating thirst, appetite, and temperature. ATP is an energy-producing molecule formed from glucose, the brain's favorite fuel source. When levels of ATP are increased in hypothalamic nerve cells, it appears that those nerve cells fire as if you had just eaten, even when you haven't.

Under Study

In the 1960s, the Bushmen disclosed the use of hoodia for appetite suppression to the South African army. The Pretoria-based CSIR then undertook animal studies with hoodia in the 1980s. The first scientific investigation of the plant was conducted at the CSIR, a partially state-funded laboratory in South Africa. Because Bushmen were known to eat hoodia, it was included in a study of indigenous foods.

Still the how and why of hoodia's use as an appetite suppressant wasn't immediately recognized. In fact, it took the laboratory thirty years to isolate and identify the specific appetite-suppressing ingredient in hoodia. "It took them a long time," said Dr. Richard Dixey during the *60 Minutes* broadcast. "In fact, the original research was done in the mid-1960s. What they found was when they fed it to animals, the animals ate it and lost weight," said Dr. Dixey.

Rights to CSIR's patent suite were then licensed to Phytopharm PLC, the UK-based botanical pharmaceutical company headed by Dixey. According to Dixey, the patent is on the active compounds within the plant and its use as a weight-loss material. "It's not on the plant itself," he said.

In 1998, Phytopharm signed a sublicensing agreement with Pfizer, allowing the pharmaceutical company to commercialize an obesity drug based on the hoodia compound. Five years later, Pfizer ended its relationship with Phytopharm. Phytopharm, which has established hoodia plantations worldwide to meet the expected demand is now looking elsewhere for a licensing partner, based not just on P57 but also on numerous semisynthetic analogs of P57 that it has produced in the interim.

In the United States, scientists at Brown University Medical School also were intrigued by the fact that P57 is chemically similar to a class of plant-derived compounds called cardiac glycosides—with ones derived from various foxglove species the best known. These powerful drugs increase the force of contraction of the heart muscle and help maintain normal heart rate and rhythm. A common side effect of the cardiac glycosides is loss of appetite.

Like many drugs, cardiac glycosides act by interacting with specific receptor molecules embedded in the walls of our cells. When stimulated by such interactions, these receptors, which are large, complex proteins that act as molecular channels, initiate a chain of events inside the cell. With cardiac glycosides, the receptor molecule is called Na/K-ATPase. Its primary function is to regulate the flow of sodium ions and potassium ions into and out of the cell through the molecular channel, using chemical energy provided by molecules of adenosine triphosphate (ATP). This process, called a sodium/potassium pump, is critically important in maintaining proper cell function and allowing cells to perform certain actions, such as muscle contraction—including of the heart muscle—and nervous impulse transmission.

Despite the similarities—including the effect of appetite suppression—between P57 and cardiac glycosides, initial studies with P57 failed to show any effect on Na/K-ATPase receptors, meaning P57 is probably not a cardiac glycoside. P57 also failed to show an effect on a wide range of other types of receptors. Thus its mode of action at the cellular level is somewhat of a mystery.

How About Humans?

The first human clinical trial conducted by Phytopharm included a group of morbidly obese men and women chosen from Leicester, England, who were placed in a prison-like phase-one unit. All the volunteers could do was read, watch television—and eat. Half the group was given hoodia and half was given a placebo. At the end of fifteen days, the group on hoodia had reduced their food intake by 1,000 calories a day. The average American man consumes about 2,600 calories a day; a woman about 1,900.

By the end of the study, those in the hoodia group had reduced their caloric intake by 30 percent, plus lost more than 2 pounds of pure body fat with no exercise—a couch potato's dream.

So far, Phytopharm has spent more than $20 million on research, including the clinical trials with obese volunteers that yielded promising results. "If you take this compound every day, your wish to eat goes down. And we've seen that very, very dramatically," said Dixey.

Research continues both in the U.S. and overseas. In two recent double-blind studies, Brown University researchers conducted experiments with normal, healthy rats in which they injected minuscule amounts of P57 directly into their brains—specifically, into a small cavity called the third intracerebral ventricle, located above the hypothalamus, which lies deep in the forebrain, just above the pituitary gland.

The purpose of these injections was to determine whether P57's appetite-suppressing effect is the result of its direct action on the hypothalamus. The researchers now believe it is. In these studies, lean and obese laboratory rats were given hoodia, which strongly suppressed their appetites and caused major weight loss in the obese rats and moderate appetite suppression and weight loss in the lean rats. Hoodia also induced a modest drop in the rats' blood sugar levels, and no adverse side effects were reported.

Specifically, the researchers found food intake was reduced by 50 to 60 percent during the first twenty-four hours after the injections, and the effect, which was dose-dependent, lasted for about twenty-four to forty-eight hours. These reductions in food intake were observed in comparison with that of a group of control rats, which had also had an inert substance injected in their brains. The researchers concluded the reductions represented a genuine effect due to P57.

They also found that injections in the abdominal cavity (intraperitoneal) of P57 did not significantly reduce the rats' food intake. This suggests that, for it to work, P57 must enter the bloodstream, which carries it to all parts of the body, including the hypothalamus.

The Brown researchers conducted additional studies on cell cultures. These studies confirmed the lack of a direct effect of P57 on the Na/K-ATPase receptors in hypothalamic cell cultures. They did find, however, that P57 did block the action of ouabain—a cardiac glycoside—on these receptors. Ouabain is a white poisonous glycoside extracted from the seeds of African trees used as a heart stimulant and by some African peoples as a dart poison.

The researchers ruled out a direct toxic effect since there has been no evidence of toxicity for P57, either in laboratory experiments or in animal studies. They decided to test for an effect of P57 on the intracellular concentration of ATP, the energy molecule that drives the sodium/potassium pump mentioned earlier.

Using a hypothalamic cell culture, they found that P57 increased the concentration of ATP by about 50 percent following a thirty-minute incubation (ouabain had no such effect). When they tested for a similar effect in live rats that were fed a normal diet, they found that brain injection with P57 increased the hypothalamic ATP levels by about 100 percent—more than twofold—compared with the controls.

The researchers then tested rats that had been on a severe low-calorie diet for four days. Without P57, these rats had hypothalamic ATP levels about 40 percent below normal (the ATP levels in their livers were about 60 percent below normal). It is reasonable to expect such decreases, because ATP is created in the body by the metabolism of food, so less food should result in less ATP—unless some other factor temporarily stimulates increased production of ATP. And that, apparently, is what P57 did, at least in the hypothalamus: when these under-fed rats were brain-injected with P57, their hypothalamic ATP levels rose to about normal, whereas the ATP levels in the control rats remained low.

In case all this scientific explanation made your eyes glaze over, suffice it to say that increased ATP production is a biochemical signal that means that you've had enough food—therefore, you don't feel hungry, so you should stop eating.

The Brown University authors did offer one caveat. Their demonstration of P57's appetite-suppressing action in the central nervous system in no way precludes the possibility that it may act to suppress appetite in other ways in other parts of the body as well, possibly through effects on the peripheral nervous system, on the stomach, or on potentially appetite-suppressing hormones, such as CCK (cholecystokinin). CCK is a kind of naturally occurring appetite-suppressing chemical. As food is digested and your body cells are "fed," CCK is released and your brain tells you to stop eating.

Some drug companies are developing cholecystokinin-booster supplements to reduce appetite in those who suffer from severe obesity. How effective these CCK boosters will be remains to be seen.

Is Hoodia Safe?

Marketers of hoodia say the most compelling evidence for the safety and efficacy of *Hoodia gordonii* as an appetite suppressant comes from its use by the Bushmen of the Kalahari for thousands of years. Nonetheless, modern pharmacologists and physicians would like to see scientific evidence for the benefits of hoodia, if only to learn how it works and how, perhaps, it could be made to work even better. So far, there have been no published clinical trials on hoodia in peer-reviewed scientific journals, although there have been unpublished reports of its efficacy by two drug companies that have been developing it for commercial purposes.

Using Hoodia

Some people say hoodia works for them immediately, suppressing appetite within twenty to thirty minutes after taking the capsules. Generally, though, people typically need up to two weeks of regularly taking hoodia before they begin to notice its effects, which include

- A reduced interest in food
- A delay in the time after eating before hunger sets in again
- Feeling full more quickly
- General feeling of well-being

BUYER BEWARE

Already, some unscrupulous companies are manufacturing a blend of cheaper ingredients with hoodia claiming that it's better than just hoodia alone. This means that you might find a product containing 1,000 mg of ingredients may have as little as 50 mg of hoodia. As a general rule, the other ingredients are only there to make the product cheaper.

All *Hoodia gordonii* supplies worldwide are the same strength. The stems of the plant are picked, dried, and milled. The powder left is about 5 percent of its original weight, which is why some quote a 20:1 extract. But don't be misled. Despite what the label may lead you to believe, you're only getting 50 mg of hoodia.

The minimum dosage to have a usable effect is around 800 to 1,200 mg (that's 800 to 1,200 mg of actual hoodia, whether you call it dried or 20:1 extract). This will help to reduce your appetite (rather than suppress it completely) so you can eat smaller meals and thus lose weight.

If you're interested in trying hoodia, look for a product that has been naturally extracted and grown or ethically wild crafted without the use of chemical fertilizers, pesticides, or preservatives; preferably in a vegetarian capsule.

Be sure it is a true standardized full-spectrum herbal supplement without fillers, binders, or common allergens.

Keep in mind that while reports of safety to date are encouraging, no significant long-term safety studies have been performed. Also, there is no data on possible drug interactions.

Hoodia is a non-stimulating herb, making it more suitable for a broader range of people, since herbal stimulants—caffeine-containing herbs such as guaraná or kola nut—can cause side effects such as elevated heart rate and blood pressure, nervousness, and sleeplessness. P57 has no sedative effects, either.

WHY IT'S HOT!

From Africa's Kalahari desert comes an exotic succulent that Bushmen have used for thousands of years to slake their thirst and curb their hunger pangs while on long hunting expeditions. This same plant—hoodia, and its derivatives—is now available in the United States as an effective appetite suppressant for those struggling with obesity or the challenge to lose additional pounds of unhealthy fat.

A compound in hoodia named P57 sends a signal to the brain, "tricking" the body into believing that it's no longer hungry and resulting in a loss of appetite. After numerous scientific studies and with an excellent safety profile, hoodia is a new—and potent—weapon in America's battle of the bulge.

HYALURONIC ACID

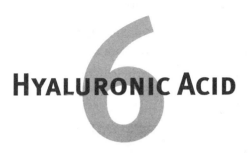

As a society, we are obsessed with youth and slowing the aging process any way we can. Methods used up to now have been primarily intrusive and cosmetic—plastic surgery, liposuction, Botox injections, etc.

Why are we so concerned with staying young and maintaining a youthful appearance? Is it because we've seen the effects of aging on our parents and others and want to age better than they did?

Did you know that more people are living longer now than at any other time in history? This is a great accomplishment, but do our bodies have a best-before-this-date stamp on our cellular makeup that determines our lifespan no matter what strategies we use to postpone the inevitability of aging? Are there ways to squeeze more quality of life from an eighty- or ninety-year-old body?

The Fountain of Youth?

What if there were a supplement that you could take that would act almost like a fountain of youth, giving you

- Younger-looking skin with fewer wrinkles
- Less-noticeable scar tissue
- Healthier, pain-free joints
- Increased immune system function
- A more youthful appearance

This is the potential of hyaluronic acid (also called hyaluronan or HA), an essential youth-maintenance material that the body manufactures in abundance during our early years but which steadily declines in quantity and quality as we age.

Discovery and Function of Hyaluronic Acid

Hyaluronic acid was first used commercially as a food source. In 1942, Endre Balazs applied for a patent to use it as a substitute for egg whites in the bakery business. I'm sure that he never dreamed how many ways it would be used.

Glycosaminoglycans (hyaluronic acid's chemical family) can be found in almost all living organisms that have joints and connective tissue. The human body is mostly made of water, and we need to keep the water content high not only in the cells but also in the tissues. This is where hyaluronic acid (HA) comes in. HA has many functions, but primarily it holds water in the tissues by binding water molecules to cells and tissue. This helps to provide the medium we need for numerous body processes and molecular transport. As with many substances found in the body, HA levels decrease as we grow older. Fifty-year-olds are estimated to have less than half as much HA as young people.

As our bodies lose the ability to hold water in tissues as we age, joint conditions such as arthritis start to appear. While arthritis is one of the more obvious symptoms of decreasing hyaluronic acid levels, another symptom of aging appears on our skin—wrinkles. Strangely enough, many of us accept joint pain and lack of mobility as a natural consequence of aging but will do all we can to reduce the appearance of wrinkles. For this reason alone, many people will use HA to supplement natural levels of glycosaminoglycans.

HYALURONIC ACID AND ITS IMPORTANCE TO HEALTH

Vanity aside, HA forms a major component of all connective tissue found in the human body. One of the functions of connective tissue is to lubricate and cushion joints. It also plays a major role in connecting the skin to the underside of tissue found everywhere in the body. When we are young, skin is elastic and able to snap back into place easily when stretched. Wrinkles are negligible because hyaluronic acid levels are high enough to maintain water levels in tissues throughout the body.

RESULTS OF COMPROMISED
HYALURONIC ACID FUNCTION

Connective tissue is found throughout the body, including areas where individuals with connective tissue disorders show the most symptoms.

Some of these connective tissue disorders include the most commonly seen chronic diseases in North America:

- TMJ
- Keratoconus
- Mitral valve prolapse
- Osteoarthritis

One thing that all these conditions have in common is that connective tissue weakness is the root cause.

The media and the general public have always been intrigued with the idea of the fountain of youth. This is apparent as we still talk about Ponce de León and his search for this fabled source of vitality and everlasting youth.

Hyaluronic acid has been called by the media the key to the fountain of youth. The ABC show "The Village of Long Life: Could Hyaluronic Acid Be an Anti-Aging Remedy?" first brought the phenomenon of hyaluronic acid to the forefront of public consciousness.

The show focused on a Japanese village where a dispro-portionate number of people live to ripe old ages—in some cases ninety years and longer. These individuals live longer and had more energy and vitality than the average American fifty years their junior. A large percentage of these seniors were incredibly healthy, vital, and strong to the extent of doing laborious tasks every day in the fields that would easily tire a person fifty years younger. What was the common denominator? Diet.

All these people ate the traditional diet, which included local root vegetables and starches that have a high nutritional content, which improves the body's natural production of HA that under normal circumstances would have declined as aging progressed.

With the increased concentration of HA throughout the tissues of these villagers, it was discovered that their skin retained its moisture, giving a much younger appearance. There were few signs of vision problems as well, and their eyes were bright and healthy. This is in spite of the fact that they worked outside in the sun every day, and in quite a few cases, they were heavy smokers all their lives—factors known to increase the aging process of skin and the body overall due to free radical generation.

Despite these facts, over 10 percent of the residents of Yuzuri Hara are eighty-five or older. This is approximately ten times the national average found in any given population in the United States. The people live longer and, more importantly, are so healthy that they rarely see a doctor and rarely succumb to chronic degenerative diseases found in the United States, such as cancer, Alzheimer's disease, and diabetes.

This widely publicized discovery eventually motivated a large Japanese pharmaceutical firm to develop the first HA supplement pills.

HYALURONIC ACID CAN AFFECT
NUMEROUS AREAS OF THE BODY

We now know many of the properties of HA and how it is used in the body.

HA is a special mucopolysaccharide that is created and used as a lubricant for human joints. It is found in substantial amounts throughout the body, especially in the young, but HA production substantially decreases as people age.

When present in a joint, even a joint with minimal or no cartilage, HA can provide a cushioning effect, reducing damage and maintaining a smooth range of motion. One of the functions of HA that gives it this property is its ability to retain and absorb up to three thousand times its own weight in water. Because of its lubricating and joint-cushioning properties, further animal studies have reported potential for disease-modifying effects and as a possible treatment for rheumatoid arthritis and osteoarthritis.

New research has revealed that HA may be able to stimulate the immune function and activate white blood cells in addition to controlling cell migration. This research indicates that HA may reduce the need for antibiotic use by stimulating the natural immune function in individuals.

In addition, HA reduces the growth rate of several strains of bacteria, and it's been reported to reduce the number of bronchitis infections in chronic patients.

As a result of its primary property of water retention and absorption, HA has now been included in cosmetic compounds such as makeup and moisturizing creams to help hold water in the skin and reduce the appearance of wrinkles.

For many years, HA has been used during cataract surgery to protect the corneal endothelium during post-operative recovery from eye surgery.

CONNECTIVE TISSUES

Connective tissue is what holds us together. It suspends and surrounds most of the organs in the body and is also involved in the delivery of nutrients to tissues and organs. There's so much connective tissue in our system, that if we removed everything else, just leaving the connective tissue, we would be able recognize ourselves in the mirror. It is not commonly known that cartilage, bone, and blood are all considered specialized forms of connective tissue. This gives some idea as to the variety of forms that connective tissue can take.

Connective tissue is also found between the cells that comprise our body. It gives our tissues substance, form, and strength. HA is an important substance in connective tissue that can be compared to the mortar that holds a brick wall together. Just as mortar is comprised of several materials including cement, sand, and water, so too is our connective tissue.

Without HA, connective tissue is severely compromised and cannot do its job properly, if at all. This is readily apparent in chronic connective tissue deficiency conditions that increase as we age.

CONSEQUENCES OF LOW HYALURONIC ACID LEVELS

With progressive aging, the body produces less hyaluronic acid, and existing hyaluronic acid breaks down more readily. Just as mortar is the first component to break down in a brick wall, collagen degradation is one of the first contributors to the primary signs of aging.

As you can see, connective tissue is involved in more than just skin formation and wrinkles! Directly or indirectly, connective tissue is critical to the pain-free and efficient functioning of almost every aspect of our body, from wound healing to skin formation and joint function.

Connective tissue disorders that have been proven to have hyaluronic acid abnormalities include

- Ehlers-Danlos Syndrome
- Marfan Syndrome
- Osteogenesis Imperfecta
- Stickler Syndrome

While these specific conditions are primarily the result of genetic damage and are often found only in certain families, these are just a few of the potential conditions involving connective tissue. In many studies on connective tissue disorders that examined hyaluronic acid, the levels were always abnormal in patients with connective tissue disorders.

Connective tissue disorders include

- Heart valve abnormality, such as mitral valve prolapse
- Joint instability
- Uncontrolled or spastic muscle contraction
- Osteoarthritis
- TMJ
- Acrogeria (premature wrinkling of the skin)
- Fibromyalgia
- Premature aging syndromes, especially Ehlers-Danlos
- Glaucoma
- Detached retinas
- Abnormal skeletal formation or hypermobility (bowed legs and double jointedness)

Hyaluronic Acid and Osteoarthritis

Hyaluronic acid levels may be another potential biomarker for osteoarthritis as we age.

It has been said that osteoarthritis will affect almost everyone if they live long enough. This degenerative joint disease is the most common form of arthritis found in our society. Once thought to be a condition of the elderly, it is now much more common at younger ages, even in teenagers.

The most common symptom of osteoarthritis is cartilage breakdown. Currently, X-rays are the most commonly used tool to diagnose osteoarthritis. Any kind of radiation, whether incidental or therapeutic, carries its own risk of free radical and radiation damage. This is not the only weakness of X-ray diagnosis. Changes in a joint may not be visible by X-ray observation for up to three years after they have occurred. This is a large window of opportunity for preemptive treatment before permanent damage occurs.

Tests that recognize the presence of biomarkers will help doctors identify early signs of disease, more reliably detect disease progression, and assess patient response to treatment. Serum hyaluronic acid levels are being studied as a potential sign of the presence and severity of osteoarthritis.

The Johnson County osteoarthritis study of 753 subjects investigated the relationship of osteoarthritis to serum HA levels. Study criteria included

- X-ray evidence of osteoarthritis
- Age
- Gender
- Race
- Body mass index (BMI)

Various self-reported coexisting disease conditions were a used as a measurement of HA levels. They included

- Circulation problems
- Cancer
- Gout
- High blood pressure
- Diabetes
- Rheumatoid arthritis

Joanne Jordan, M.D., M.P.H., and her colleagues at the University of North Carolina–Chapel Hill and Duke University, reported that there was a strong association between serum HA levels and an increasing severity of osteoarthritis as measured by X-rays of the knees and hips. Additionally, regardless of disease severity, serum HA was generally higher in men compared to women, and in Caucasians compared to African Americans.

Only gout was found to have an independent association with serum HA, possibly as a result of the severe inflammation and joint damage caused by gout.

One surprising aspect of this study was that gender and ethnicity played a role in HA production and levels. More research is needed to explore what underlies the finding of higher serum HA levels in men and in Caucasians.

DIFFERENT FORMS OF HYALURONIC ACID

Much of the research on HA has been done on injectable forms; the HA is injected directly into the affected joints to increase mobility and reduce pain. Most, but not all, studies reported good results using this method.

Some of the varied results of this research are outlined below.

Osteoarthritis of the knee affects up to 10 percent of the elderly population. The condition is frequently treated by intra-articular injection of HA. A systematic review and meta-analysis of randomized controlled trials has been initiated to assess the effectiveness of this treatment.

Twenty-two different studies were identified and included in this review of the efficacy of hyaluronic acid injection an osteoarthritic knees. Measurement of symptoms such as level of pain at rest, during or immediately after movement, joint function, and adverse side effects were all included. The end result was that pain at rest was reduced by HA injection.

Despite the improvement reported, this report suggests that HA has not been fully proven to be clinically effective and suggests that larger trials are necessary to further discover the benefits and risks of HA injection.

One study reported that patients experience better results from HA injections if they have milder forms of OA or if they start treatment earlier. The later HA therapy is started and the more advanced the joint damage is, the less effective HA will be.

As OA advances, the joint space becomes narrower until bone rests on bone with no cartilage left for cushioning. The primary objective of another study was to investigate structural changes, as measured by joint space narrowing (JSN), within the knee joint during treatment with intra-articular injection of HA of molecular weight 500–730 kDa in patients with osteoarthritis of the knee.

This double-blind human study included the use of regular weekly injections of either HA or placebo over three weeks. Treatment with pain medications was allowed. The only measurement of success or failure was the reduction in the joint space width or joint space narrowing (JSN). A total of 408 patients were randomized and 319 completed the one-year study.

In patients with radiologically more severe disease, there was no difference in JSN between the two treatments. Although, in this one-year study, no overall treatment effect was seen, those with radiologically milder disease at the start of the study had less progression of joint space narrowing when treated with hyaluronic acid.

In a third study, individuals who had never used HA injections were investigated.

These patients received a series of three injections over a period of three weeks. The results differed greatly from the previous studies. Researchers reported that HA injections were very effective in reducing overall arthritic pain and were highly effective in reducing resting and walking pain after the first and a second treatment series. The patients were very satisfied with the therapy and had very few local adverse events.The therapeutic effect typically lasted six months. Reduced use of other pain-reduction modalities including drug therapy for pain was also reported. These data support the potential role of intra-articular hyaluronic acid as an effective long-term therapeutic option for patients with osteoarthritis of the knee.

The Holy Grail of HA research for many years has been to find a topical or oral application that is easily absorbed by the human body. Previously published studies have reported that topical and oral HA are not easily absorbed and therefore do not create the needed increase in serum HA levels. But new research has reported that an orally administered form of HA has been discovered that demonstrates significant absorption and bioavailability in normal volunteer subjects.

A recent clinical study published in the *FASEB Journal* confirms that sternal hydrolyzed collagen type II combined with hyaluronic acid is safe and effective in relieving pain and stiffness as a result of osteoarthritis and promotes joint health in adults.

Until now, regular or native collagen (which has not been predigested but does contain HA) consisting of giant molecules that were much too large for easy absorption in the human digestive tract was the only format available.

The key to increase the absorption was to reduce the typical molecular weight of collagen and HA. Reducing the molecular weight to between 1,500 and 2,500 Daltons substantially increases absorption and bioavailability .

By determining the rate and level of HA absorption and its bioavailability in the body, this study clearly demonstrates that this specific type of HA has the physical characteristics necessary to allow it and its metabolites to move rapidly from the blood to the tissues, where it can provide therapeutic reduction of symptoms.

The Federation of American Societies for Experimental Biology recently released clinical research results on oral delivery of radio-labeled hyaluronan and its ability to be utilized by joints. Dr. Alex Schauss, director of the American Institute for Biosocial and Medical Research, presented the findings at the FASEB's 2004 conference. The study proved that HA can be absorbed effectively through the intestine and increase serum HA levels, especially if the molecules are small enough.

Until now, there were no data on absorption levels for orally administered HA. As a result, the therapeutic use of

HA was limited to injections or topical applications. The results of this study, which examined the absorption, excretion, and distribution of radio-labeled HA after a single oral administration in genetically modified Wistar rats and Beagle dogs, demonstrated that HA is absorbed and distributed to organs and joints after even a single oral administration.

This research is some of the earliest that suggests that hyaluronic acid can be absorbed from oral administration, which paves the way for HA dietary supplements to treat osteoarthritis.

Why It's Hot!

Hyaluronic acid, though still in its infancy after being studied for over thirty years, is proving to be a valuable ally in the treatment of several conditions. Osteoarthritis and skin conditions all responded well to HA. The fact that it has few, if any, side effects and offers long-lasting therapeutic results makes it a natural addition to any baby boomer's medicine cabinet.

Reminder

HA is hydrophilic (water loving) and can capture up to three thousand times its own weight in water to act as a lubricant and cushion for joints. HA can't live up to this potential if you are dehydrated. It's crucial to drink half your body weight in ounces. If you weigh 150 pounds, drink a minimum of 75 ounces per day on an empty stomach.

7

MANGOSTEEN

What has long been a favored fruit throughout the tropical world is now being discovered as a drink and a dietary supplement in the United States. Mangosteen juice and supplements are marketed as a source of energy and antioxidants that help boost the immune system and slow the aging process. There are also claims that it can cure cancer, improve blood circulation, strengthen the immune system, and lead to a long, healthy life. While many benefits are being attributed to mangosteen, what are the facts?

A MANGOSTEEN ISN'T A MANGO

Mangoes and mangosteens may have similar names, but they don't bear any resemblance to each other, and botanically they belong to different species. The mango is from the species *Mangifera*, with closer ties to cashews and pistachios, while the *mangosteen (Garcinia mangostana L.)* is from the *Clusiaceae* family and *Garcinia* species. The species *Garcinia* contains some three hundred members growing throughout the tropical areas of the world from Asia to the Caribbean. It is cousin to *Garcinia cambogia*, a source of hydroxycitric acid (HCA), which is found in many weight-loss products.

Unlike mango trees, which grow in Southern California and Florida, the mangosteen is virtually unknown in the United States because it cannot grow here despite attempts to do so. One reference claims that a mangosteen tree grew in Florida, produced one fruit, and promptly died. It is a very slow-growing tree that flourishes in wet lowland tropical climates with lots of humidity to protect it from the sun, and heat to protect it from cold (it dies at temperatures below 41 degrees Fahrenheit).

Nor is its fruit found fresh in supermarkets. One can find it canned in Asian markets, but it isn't equal in flavor to the fresh fruit that must be picked ripe, has no lasting power, and bruises easily. Yet devotees say that once you've tasted a fresh mangosteen fruit, its delicate flavor is memorable yet difficult to describe—the flavors of peach, banana, grape, apple, and pineapple have all been ascribed to the mangosteen.

WHAT'S FOOD AND WHAT'S MEDICINE?

The mangosteen is a small, firm fruit that's the size and shape of a medium tomato. It has a deep eggplant-purple skin. Slice it open around its middle and you'll find a deep red pericarp (thick rind), about 1/2 inch thick, which protects the succulent white segmented fruit and black seeds at its heart. It is these white, pulpy segments, five to eight in number, that are eaten. The spongy, deep red, astringent pericarp is usually discarded. The delicious white segments, however, are not the part of the fruit that contains all of the potent antioxidants, but they are rich in phytin, an organic phosphorus compound.

Fruits that are rich in polyphenolic antioxidants are usually deep red, blue, or purple, like the mangosteen's pericarp. Although the pectin-rich pericarp has been made into an edible purple jelly in some countries, it is so astringent that it must first be soaked in a 6 percent brine solution to reduce its 7–14 percent catechin and tannin content.

The unsavory pericarp also contains a wealth of other medicinal compounds that are of interest to researchers. Apart from its catechins and tannins, it is reputed to contain one of the highest sources of xanthones, phenolic plant compounds that are being researched for their anti-tumor, antibacterial, and fungicidal properties. It is the dried and powdered pericarp that has traditionally been used medicinally in Singapore, India, and China.

Free Radicals: Bad Boys of the Atomic World

Electrons are negatively charged particles that circle around the outer shell of atoms, much like planets circle around the sun. They usually come in pairs. Atoms might share their electron pairs with other atoms, thereby binding

the atoms into larger molecules, which then bond together to form cells, which then clump into tissue, muscle,
nerves, and bone.

Electrons also incite chemical reactions. When an oxygen atom has paired electrons, it is stable. When it loses an
electron, it becomes a free radical. A free radical is unstable and reacts by trying to steal an electron from another
oxygen atom to regain its stability. If it succeeds, the other
atom becomes unstable and starts a chain reaction when it
too tries to take an electron away from another atom. This
can start a cascading effect until the entire molecule, the
DNA, the cell, and larger tissue is damaged. If the cell's
DNA—the molecules that provide chemical instructions
to the cell—is damaged, the entire cell can die. Free radicals are partially responsible for the aging process and are
suspected of contributing to the development of various
diseases.

What causes this to happen? Cells continuously produce free radicals as they go about their daily business. The
oxygen you breathe gives you life, but it also causes oxidation, which forms free radicals that produce oxidative
stress. Oxidation causes the lipid-based components of
your cells and tissues to become rancid and the water-
based components to form toxins (hydrogen peroxide and
other reactive oxygen species [ROS]). Metabolic processes—even your own body's immune system—produce free
radicals as they fight invading bacteria and viruses. This
can start a chain reaction, which if not halted by antioxidant activity, can cause disease or death at the cellular level.

External factors, such as environmental pollutants, radiation, chemicals, and smoke also contribute to our daily free radical burden. With a good diet and healthy lifestyle, our bodies can protect and repair themselves, but as we age, we accumulate an overwhelming burden of free radical damage that cannot be repaired by the antioxidants we consume. A lifetime of poor nutrition, tobacco use, and excessive alcohol consumption only accelerates the aging process.

Some of the most common free radical terms you might encounter are:

- Reactive Singlet Oxygen Species (ROS): Any free radical involving oxygen atoms
- Lipid Peroxidation: The result of a free-radical attack on a cell lipid (fat) membrane, cholesterol, or any polyunsaturated lipid molecules found in the body
- Hydroxyl Radicals: The most damaging free radical in the body, it is produced continuously by the combination of dioxide (O_2) and hydrogen peroxide (H_2O_2)
- Hydrogen Peroxide: Produces hydroxyl radicals or can be converted to water (H_2O)

These are but a few common free radicals involving hydrogen and oxygen molecules; there are many more. Free radical damage has been implicated in Parkinson's disease, Alzheimer's disease, as well as various cancers and cardiovascular conditions.

Antioxidants: Coming to the Rescue!

Antioxidants neutralize, or "quench," free radicals by donating electrons to them so they become stable.

Antioxidants come in many forms—certain vitamins, minerals, amino acids, and some enzymes have this capacity. Most plants contain a variety of these antioxidant compounds, but they also contain a special category of antioxidants called polyphenols, which contribute a great deal of antioxidant activity to the body.

Some antioxidants work in a lipid (fat) environment and others work in a water environment. Since cells throughout the body contain both water and lipid components, taking a variety of both water-soluble and fat-soluble antioxidants is a two-pronged approach to providing the body with the right kinds and amounts of antioxidants needed. Antioxidants also have the added benefit that they help each other regenerate their antioxidant potential by recycling electrons among themselves.

Antioxidants are found primarily in fresh fruits and vegetables, as well as dietary supplements.

The Pucker Factor

The mangosteen pericarp is rich in tannins, which are a group of phenols that can make your mouth pucker as they provide astringency to various foods such as unripe grapes, persimmons, and blueberries. Tannins are a defense mechanism that plants use to ward off predators until the seeds of the fruits are ripe. Tea is high in tannins, as are red wine and dark chocolate. But while a small amount of tannins produces a pleasant bite and enhance flavor, too much can be unpleasant, which is why the mangosteen pericarp, with its very high tannin content is not usually eaten as a food. Tannins, however, do have certain health benefits—they help increase saliva production, and they have been shown to decrease appetite by binding to proteins, starch, and cellulose, which enhances a feeling of satiety.

If you want all the benefits of the pericarp xanthone and antioxidants in a juice, it must be blended with other mangosteen juices, or with a combination of different juice concentrates (apple, cherry, pomegranate, to name a few) to offset its astringency. Or, if you want a product with all of the goodness and none of the taste of the pericarp, the dried powder can be found in capsule form in dietary supplements at your health food stores.

ANTIAGING ANTIOXIDANTS

Pick up any magazine or newspaper today and you'll find articles that link free radical damage to aging. The key, many claim, to halting, or at least slowing, the aging process is to eat plenty of fruits and vegetables, so there will be sufficient antioxidants to fight against accumulating free radicals.

Mangosteen contains several types of antioxidants, consisting mainly of catechins and some vitamin C (ascorbic acid) and beta-carotene, both of which are well known for their antioxidant properties.

Vitamin C is a water-soluble vitamin that helps quench reactive singlet oxygen species (oxygen atoms that have lost an electron—see Free Radicals above). Beta-carotene is a fat-soluble vitamin that is common in all red, orange, and yellow vegetables and fruits. It is the most studied carotenoid, and it also helps quench singlet oxygen species.

Catechins are not vitamins, they are plant polyphenols, but they have a similar antioxidant activity. In the same category as tannins, they fall into a different subcategory of flavonols. Catechins have found their claim to fame in green tea. They are also found in abundance in grapes, wine, and chocolate. The pericarp of the mangosteen is extremely rich in catechins. An average mangosteen pericarp contains approximately 50–60 mg of catechins, about the same as found in 100 grams of dark chocolate.

The antioxidant capacity of plants hasn't been measured until recently. But now, a new designation, ORAC (Oxygen Radical Absorbance Capacity), is starting to be used on fruits in supermarkets and antioxidant supplements in health food stores. Mangosteen supplements and juices are some of the first products to use this measurement of antioxidant capacity.

ORAC

Recently, assays have been developed that can measure the amount of peroxyl radical–scavenging antioxidants in a given fruit or vegetable in ORAC units. The higher the ORAC value, the greater the antioxidant activity. While the average person consumes about 1,200 ORAC units per day, research suggests that people should consume between 3,000 and 5,000 ORAC units daily for optimal health. Five hundred milligrams of pericarp powder typically contains approximately 1,500–1,700 ORAC units.

XANTHONES: PROMISING SUPERHEROES

Xanthones also belong to the polyphenol family, and although much of the antioxidant activity of various members of this large family has been explored and explained, xanthones are still a bit of a mystery because more research needs to be conducted. Several members of the xanthone family have been identified. In this family, many members have been given Greek-letter prefixes (like some vitamins), of which the most studied are the alpha-, beta-, and gamma-mangostins, as well as simple mangostin, and various methoxyxanthones. Mangostin has been shown to inhibit the oxidation of LDL cholesterol, which is implicated in plaque formation in arteries (arteriosclerosis). Mangostin's health benefits also include antibacterial and fungicidal properties, and, most promising of all, antitumor activities.

WHAT DOES THE RESEARCH SAY?

Most mangosteen studies have focused on its xanthones. Although xanthones have some antioxidant properties in support of good health, researchers worldwide have been more interested in exploring their pharmaceutical potential to treat severe illnesses. While preliminary research has been in vitro, if current studies show promise more research will be needed on animals and humans.

Several studies on six xanthones from the pericarp of the mangosteen have been conducted in vitro to determine if the xanthones inhibited the growth of human leukemia cells and cancerous liver cells. Both studies have demonstrated great success in killing the cancer cells, which suggests that alpha-mangostin and its cohorts might be potential candidates for eventual preventative and therapeutic cancer treatments.

Another in vitro study tested the antibacterial activity of some xanthones on antibiotic-resistant *Staphylococcus aureus* bacteria and shows promising pharmaceutical applications. Still another study appears to show in vitro activity against tuberculosis.

Why It's Hot!

As an antioxidant, mangosteen heads the top of the list! With more and more baby boomers hitting fifty, the emphasis today is on active lifestyles, maintaining good health, and living longer. To do this, more and more people are turning to dietary supplementation with a variety of antioxidants. Even with the latest food pyramid, it can be difficult to get all the antioxidants we need from our diets. Drinking mangosteen juice, or taking mangosteen pericarp capsules, can give us a powerhouse of tannins, catechins, and xanthones that we need to arm our body with enough antioxidants to help minimize the free radicals waging cellular combat inside our bodies.

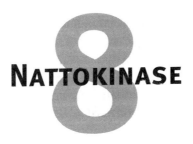

NATTOKINASE

Nattokinase is an enzyme that has been present in the Japanese food *natto* for thousands of years and which recent studies have shown to have anticoagulant properties. But we can't really talk about nattokinase without talking about how fortunate you are to not have to eat natto anymore to reap the benefits. To the uninitiated, natto is scary. It's a traditional Japanese dish of fermented soybeans that has been a staple in the Japanese diet for thousands of years.

Exactly how many thousands of years cannot be determined, but the items required to make natto—beans, straw, water, and time—have been available in Japan for centuries. Natto is made by soaking soybeans in water for up to a day, then steaming the beans for several hours and finally mixing the beans with a sauce and rice straw and allowing it to ferment for twenty-four hours.

The magic of natto takes place when the bacterium *Bacillus natto*, present on the rice straw, is combined with the soybeans. This is how nattokinase is born. Without the bacterium, natto would be just another bowl of stinky beans.

An important development in the history of natto was when, in the early twentieth century, researchers discovered a way to introduce *Bacillus natto* into the soybean mix without using straw, therefore simplifying the process of making natto and producing more consistent results.

Its sticky appearance and strong odor—if you like blue cheese you'll like natto!—are an acquired taste, and even in Japan natto is mostly eaten only in the eastern region of Kanto.

USDA nutritional information states that natto is "very low in cholesterol and sodium. It is also a good source of protein, Vitamin K, magnesium and copper, and a very good source of iron and manganese."

As a good source of vitamin K, natto contributes to the formation of calcium-binding groups in proteins, assisting the formation of bone and preventing osteoporosis. Vitamin K1 is found naturally in seaweed, liver, and some vegetables, while vitamin K2 is found in fermented food products like cheese and miso. Natto has very large amounts of vitamin K2.

Japanese pets have also enjoyed natto as an ingredient in their food and it has allegedly improved their health. The animals also don't seem to mind natto's smell and sliminess.

In spite of its smell and appearance, natto has a surprisingly mild taste and has been used in Japan for years as a folk remedy to treat heart and vascular diseases as well as fatigue and beriberi.

NATTO AS A MODERN REMEDY

The scope and degree of the benefits of nattokinase were not documented until fairly recently. Its potent thrombolytic activity is what's currently gaining nattokinase attention and credibility.

Japanese researcher Dr. Hiroyuki Sumi studied thrombolytic enzymes while at the University of Chicago Medical School majoring in physiological chemistry. He wanted to find a natural enzyme that would help dissolve blood clots associated with heart attacks and strokes.

In 1980, Dr. Sumi tested over 173 natural foods as part of his research. You can imagine his joy when he dropped natto in a petri dish on fibrin (a protein that forms in the blood to stop excess blood loss after trauma or injury and is chemically similar to thrombus) and within eighteen hours the natto had completely dissolved the fibrin.

Heart disease and stroke are the first and third causes of death in the United States. They account for more deaths than all the cancers and injuries combined. To have discovered a supplement that originates from a natural source, has already been used for thousands of years, and has a number of additional benefits—including lowering blood pressure—is a great leap forward in the quest to prevent cardiovascular disease.

INTRODUCTION TO FIBRIN

Fibrin is a natural protein in our blood. When strands of fibrin accumulate in our blood vessels, blood clots form. Individual strands of fibrin are always present, but they undergo a chemical change and will stick together to form a blood clot as the body's natural response to injury or trauma. This clotting process is a vital function, but problems occur when a body is unable to completely break down the clots once they have served their purpose.

The body produces more than twenty enzymes to produce blood clots, but only makes one to get rid of them. Plasmin is the body's natural enzyme for breaking down blood clots. If not enough plasmin is produced, then the blood clots are not completely dissolved and the pieces will flow through the bloodstream, damaging blood vessel linings and sometimes blocking blood vessels completely.

A blood clot can block the flow of blood to muscle tissue. Blood carries oxygen, and if that oxygen supply is cut off, the tissue will eventually die. In the heart, a blood clot can result in angina and heart attacks. A blood clot in the chambers of the heart can then move to the brain. A blood clot that stops the flow of blood through the brain leads to senility and/or stroke.

Aging patients are the most likely to benefit from the blood-thinning effects of nattokinase. As the body ages, plasmin production declines, making the blood more likely to coagulate leading to cardiac and cerebral infarction. Nattokinase's ability to improve circulatory health will affect those who suffer from conditions resulting from arteries clogged by blood clots, that is, patients with senile dementia whose cerebral arteries were blocked.

Nattokinase is a natural enzyme that complements the body's natural production of plasmin. It is capable of potently dissolving fibrin as well as activating the prourokinase pathways to stimulate the body to produce its own plasmin. This complementary ability works in contrast to current pharmaceutical drugs, which can interfere with the normal clotting process. Most drugs are formulated to inhibit platelet aggregation, or the blood's ability to clot. Nattokinase, on the other hand, seems to clean up old blood clots that would otherwise circulate through the bloodstream and cause damage to blood vessels.

"In all my years of research as a professor of cardiovascular and pulmonary medicine, natto and nattokinase represent the most exciting new development in the prevention and treatment of cardiovascular-related diseases," said Dr. Martin Milner of the Center for Natural Medicine in Portland. Dr. Milner and Dr. Kouhei Makise of Kyoto, Japan, collaborated on a research project on nattokinase and wrote an extensive paper on their findings.

"We have finally found a potent natural agent that can thin and dissolve clots effectively, and with relative safety and without side effects," said Dr. Milner.

RISK FACTORS FOR CARDIOVASCULAR DISEASE

Risk factors are traits that are used to measure a person's likelihood to develop a disease. The more risk factors you have, the greater your risk. While many factors are hereditary, there are many on this list over which you have control.

- High cholesterol
- Family history
- High blood pressure
- Overweight
- Smoking
- Physical inactivity

TIPS TO REDUCE YOUR RISK OF CARDIOVASCULAR DISEASE

- Stop smoking!
- Exercise
- Eat a diet rich in whole-grain foods and fiber
- Drink eight to ten glasses of water per day
- Regular resistance training/muscle strength training
- Practice a stress-reduction technique

RESEARCH

To date, seventeen studies have been devoted to natto and nattokinase, including two human trials. In 1990, Dr. Sumi and his research team published a series of reports on their findings of the clot-dissolving properties of nattokinase.

In the latest human study, researchers from JCR Pharmaceuticals, Oklahoma State University, and Miyazaki Medical College tested nattokinase on twelve healthy

Japanese volunteers—six women and six men between the ages of twenty-one and fifty-five. The volunteers were given 7 ounces of natto before breakfast, and researchers then tracked fibrinolytic activity (or breakdown of fibrin) through a series of blood tests.

In one test, a blood sample was taken and a clot was artificially induced. The amount of time needed to dissolve the clot was cut in half within two hours of treatment, compared to the control group. The volunteers also retained an ability to dissolve blood clots for up to eight hours.

On average, the volunteers' ELT (a measure of how long it takes to dissolve a blood clot) dropped by 48 percent within two hours of treatment.

The control group in the study ate only boiled soybeans and their blood tests showed no significant fibrinolytic activity.

Dr. Sumi's team conducted a test on two groups of dogs: one group received nattokinase tablets and the other group received a placebo. The team then created a clot in a major leg vein in each dog that completely blocked the vein. Within five hours, the nattokinase-fed dogs had a complete restoration of circulation in their leg veins, while the dogs fed the placebo still had a complete vein blockage eighteen hours later.

Researchers from Biotechnology Research Laboratories and JCR Pharmaceuticals Company of Kobe, Japan, tested nattokinase's ability to dissolve a blood clot in the carotid arteries of rats. Animals treated with nattokinase regained 62 percent of blood flow compared with those treated with plasmin that only regained 15.8 percent of blood flow.

And finally, in another laboratory study, endothelial (the inner lining of blood vessels) damage was induced in the femoral arteries of rats that had been given nattokinase. In normal circumstances, a thickening of arterial walls and blood clotting would occur, but they were both suppressed because of nattokinase's fibrinolytic activity.

BLOOD PRESSURE

Although used as a traditional folk medicine in Japan to treat high blood pressure, recent studies confirm this benefit of nattokinase. In 1995, the effects of nattokinase on high blood pressure was studied in both animals and humans at Japan's Miyazaki Medical College and Kurashiki University of Science and Arts.

RESEARCH

Volunteers with high blood pressure were given 30 grams of natto extract (equivalent to 7 ounces of natto food), for four days. In four out of five volunteers, their systolic blood pressure dropped about 10.9 percent on the average, and their diastolic blood pressure dropped about 9.7 percent on the average.

Rats that were given natto extract showed an average decrease on blood pressure after just two hours. The data showed an approximate 12.7 percent drop in systolic blood pressure.

Nattokinase is particularly potent because it enhances the body's natural ability to fight blood clots in several different ways, said Dr. Milner.

"In some ways, nattokinase is actually superior to conventional clot-dissolving drugs," said Dr. Milner. "T-PAs (tissue plasminogen activators) like urokinase (the drug), are only effective when taken intravenously and often fail simply because a stroke or heart-attack victim's arteries have been hardened beyond the point where they can be treated by any other clot-dissolving agent. Nattokinase, however, can help prevent that hardening."

RETINAL VEIN OCCLUSION

A team of researchers decided to use nattokinase in a case study to treat a retinal vein occlusion. In other words, the blood vessels draining out of the eye of a fifty-eight-year-old man were blocked by a blood clot. The blockage had caused bleeding in the eye and swelling from by the backed-up blood, resulting in tiny vessels bursting. Using natto as the source of nattokinase, researchers fed the man a 100-gram serving before going to bed every night. Ten days later, the bleeding from the bottom of his eye was stopped. And at twenty days, the man's vision was recovered and he was sent home from the hospital with instructions to continue to eat natto twice a week. In the space of two months, the nattokinase had completely dissolved the occlusion.

Cholesterol

Recent research indicates that the body's natural response to an injury by blood clots to arterial walls is to build up cholesterol in arterial plaques. Hence, if nattokinase can prevent blood clots from forming in the blood, then heightened cholesterol levels could be avoided.

Diabetes

Certain types of diabetes have also been shown to be due to changes in the blood vessels supplying the pancreas, again tied to small blood clots in these vessels.

Forms and Dosage

As mentioned earlier, natto is the original form and source of nattokinase. However, thanks to modern technology, nattokinase is available in capsule form. A wide range and variety is currently available, including a highly advanced supplement that contains no soy and no vitamin K.

The standard dosage recommendations are 2,000 FU (fibrin units—or 50 grams) daily for a preventative, and 4,000 to 6,000 FU (160 to 200 grams) daily for therapeutic use.

For those using nattokinase for therapeutic purposes, it's important to use a high-quality, researched nattokinase enzyme standardized for potency and guaranteed to be free of vitamin K to prevent bleeding side effects and contraindications.

DRUG INTERACTIONS AND SIDE EFFECTS

Natto is considered a safe traditional food when eaten in moderate amounts. However, nattokinase enzyme and extracts that naturally contain vitamin K can interfere with blood-thinning drugs like coumadin and aspirin. Therefore, patients who are currently on blood thinners and those who suffer from kidney or liver disease should consult their doctor before using nattokinase.

People with bleeding disorders, such as hemophilia or a group of diseases called hermorrhagic diathesias, should not take nattokinase. People with ongoing bleeding problems, including ulcers, recent surgery, or recent major trauma should also avoid taking nattokinase.

Pregnant or nursing women should consult their doctors before using nattokinase until additional research confirms its safety.

WHY IT'S HOT!

Though it's stinky and slimy in its natural state, the fermented soy product nattokinase has demonstrated some prettty remarkable health-promoting qualities in clinical research. Chief among them is nattokinase's ability to improve circulatory health through its blood-thinning and anticlotting properties. With heart disease and stroke the number-one and number-three killers in the United States, nattokinase may prove to be a significant addition to the arsenal of disease-preventing supplements now available at your local health food store.

OMEGA-3 FATTY ACIDS

We've been hearing all kinds of conflicting information about fats over the past few years: First, all fats were bad, and experts sang the praises of a low-fat diet, telling us to limit all sources of dietary fat as much as possible. Then there was the high-fat, high-protein Atkins diet craze, which found followers breakfasting on as much bacon and eggs as they liked and shunning all forms of carbohydrates. But recent studies have shown that it's not necessarily how much fat you eat that will most influence your health, but rather what kinds of fat.

Researchers have recently noted that people who follow the traditional Mediterranean diet, which is not necessarily low in fat but which emphasizes olive oil and fish as primary sources of fat, suffer fewer incidences of heart disease. Likewise, the traditional diet of the Inuit centers on cold-water marine mammals such as whales and seals, animals that are very rich in saturated fat. However, these creatures are also abundant sources of omega-3 fatty acids, a valuable nutrient that has most likely contributed to the low rates of cardiovascular disease among the Inuit in the past.

WHAT ARE ESSENTIAL FATTY ACIDS?

Essential fatty acids are fats that play vital structural and regulatory roles in the body. There are two kinds of essential fatty acids: omega-3 and omega-6. (Their names derive from the system of chemical notation used to describe molecules.) The human body needs saturated fatty acids (SFAs), monounsaturated fatty acids (MUFAs), and polyunsaturated fatty acids (PUFAs) in order to thrive and even survive. We can make the other fats we need from the food we eat, but we lack the enzymes to synthesize omega-3 and omega-6 (both PUFAs). We must get these fats from our diet.

Omega-6 fatty acids are plentiful in nature, occurring in many seeds, nuts, and oils, including vegetable oils such as corn, safflower, and sunflower. On the other hand, omega-3s occur in only a few plants that humans eat, including flax seeds, hemp seeds, pumpkin seeds, walnuts, purslane, and canola and soy oil (this plant-based variety of omega-3 is called alpha linolenic acid). Omega-3s are, however, abundant in plants that wild fish and animals eat, such as algae and wild grasses.

Our prehistoric forebears ate fish, fowl, and mammals that had fed on these wild grasses and algae. The fat of these creatures was rich in omega-3s from these grasses and algae (this is the other variety of omega-3, called docosahexaenoic acid and eicosapentaenoic acid). The fat of these animals was also abundant in omega-6s, and as a result, our ancestors' diets were full of both omega-3 fatty acids and omega-6 fatty acids. Researchers think the Paleolithic diet contained omega-6s and omega-3s in about equal proportions.

In contrast, today's farm-raised animals are generally fed grains such as corn that provide omega-6s but not omega-3s. Additionally, people today tend to consume a lot of their fat in the form of vegetable oils and margarines that are high in omega-6s but not omega-3s. Scientists estimate the ratio of omega-6 fatty acids to omega-3s in the modern diet ranges between twenty to one and forty to one, an imbalance that may be causing heart disease, cancer, and autoimmune diseases. Some researchers postulate an ideal ratio of three (omega-6s) to one (omega-3s).

IMPORTANCE OF ESSENTIAL FATTY ACIDS

Essential fatty acids play a key role in the synthesis of crucial hormones called prostaglandins. These hormones oversee cell growth and differentiation, immune function, and blood clotting. Prostaglandins can either strengthen or weaken the body's inflammation response, and they can intensify or reduce blood clotting.

Prostaglandins that come from omega-6 fatty acids tend to encourage inflammation and blood clotting, and those made from omega-3 fatty acids tend to counter these effects. As with so many things in nature and in our bodies, these two opposing forces must strike a balance to maintain vibrant health. Since the modern Western diet is skewed toward an overabundance of omega-6s, either inclusion of more cold-water fish and flax seeds in the diet or supplementation with omega-3s is a must.

Benefits of Omega-3 Supplementation

Fish oil containing omega-3s can be helpful in lowering triglyceride levels, reducing the risk of death from coronary heart disease, decreasing blood clotting, lowering blood pressure, alleviating symptoms of rheumatoid arthritis and ulcerative colitis, preventing relapses of Crohn's disease, reducing dysmenorrhea, lessening depression, and stabilizing moods in bipolar disorder.

Here's a quick overview of some of the research that has been done:

An analysis of the myriad trials investigating omega-3s vis-à-vis heart disease shows that a high intake of fish or fish oil can decrease death due to heart disease and sudden cardiac death. Fish oils have been shown to reduce serum triglycerides and may even raise HDL levels a modest amount (HDL is the "good cholesterol"). Higher dietary consumption of omega-3s may reduce incidence of cardiovascular disease.

Thirteen different studies involving a total of more than five hundred individuals found that fish oils can reduce symptoms of rheumatoid arthritis (however, fish oils don't seem to slow disease progression).

Two different studies in women have shown that daily supplementation with fish oil results in significantly diminished menstrual pain.

Individuals with bipolar disorder experienced longer symptom-free periods when they were taking fish oil capsules, and one study showed that people with recurrent depression improved with use of omega-3s.

WHY IT'S HOT!

Research into the health-promoting effects of omega-3s is ongoing, but enough studies have already been done to demonstrate how crucial these essential fatty acids are. Whether you opt to feast on wild Alaskan salmon, sprinkle ground flax seeds on your cereal, or take one of the many fish oil capsules available, you're taking an important step toward ensuring your overall health and well-being.

POSSIBLE SIDE EFFECTS

Rare interactions can occur between fish oil supplements and aspirin, garlic, and ginkgo. Due to the blood-thinning activity of omega-3s, increased bleeding time may occur, as well as more frequent nosebleeds and easy bruising. Do not take if you have a bleeding disorder or are on anticoagulants. Do not take if you are allergic to fish. Diabetics should consult with their physicians before taking omega-3s.

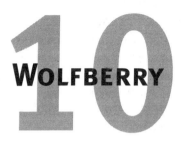

WOLFBERRY

Used for its many healing properties for thousands of years in China, the wolfberry (goji berry; *Lycium barbarum; Gou Qi Zi;* or *Ningxia* wolfberry) has been rediscovered in the West, and its amazing antioxidant and health benefits are now available to all.

HISTORY OF THE WOLFBERRY

Considered a treasure for generations in China, Chinese physicians have studied the medicinal properties of the wolfberry since before the Tang Dynasty (ca. 800 A.D.). A poem from that time describes a well situated next to a wall near a Buddhist temple. The wall was covered with wolfberry vines, and the berries fell into the well and mixed with the water that the locals drank. Due to the remarkable rejuvenative qualities of this "wolfberry water," eighty-year-old men and women were reported to have maintained radiant complexions, dark hair, and healthy teeth and gums.

Though this story is apocryphal, many sources, including a Chinese Medica dating back over two thousand years, recommend eating wolfberries to strengthen and restore the major organ systems and replenish the qi, or vital life-force. Another Chinese medical text, written by Shen Nung Ben Tsao (475–221 B.C.), also extolled the benefits of the wolfberry for the major body systems and qi. Writing in a physician's handbook from the Ming Dynasty (1368–1644 A.D.), Ben Cao Gang Mu said that, "taking in Chinese wolfberry regularly may regulate the flow of vital energy and strengthen the physique, which can lead to longevity." In fact, the ancient Chinese revered three medicinal herbs above all others: ling tzi, ginseng, and the wolfberry.

Health benefits of wolfberries cited by ancient Chinese texts include:

- Enhances the qi (or life-force)
- Improves vision
- Supports the kidneys and liver
- Acts as a blood tonic
- Nourishes the yin
- Strengthens bones and muscles

BOTANICAL PROPERTIES OF THE WOLFBERRY

A member of the *Solanaceae* (or nightshade) family—along with potatoes, tomatoes, and tobacco—wolfberries grow on a wild bush that's native to the northwest region of China. The wolfberry plant can tolerate temperatures ranging from –27 degrees Celsius to 39 degrees Celsius. A bushy perennial plant, the wolfberry typically grows to a height of 3–5 feet, with narrow 2-inch-long spear-shaped leaves and flowers ranging from light purple to blue. The flowers are hermaphrodites (with male and female organs) and are pollinated by bees. It takes from four to five years from seeding until the plants begin bearing fruit. When fully ripe, the red berries are oblong in shape and plump with juice. This full size, red color, and sweet taste are hallmarks of the wolfberry.

Blooming from April to October, wolfberries are harvested between June and October depending on geography and weather. Because the berries are so tender when ripe and will oxidize when touched, they cannot be hand picked. Instead the vines must be shaken, with the berries falling gently onto collection mats. The ripe berries are then preserved in a slow process of drying, sometimes in the shade and sometimes in the sun. Once dried, the berries are about the size of raisins and taste like a cross between a cranberry and a cherry.

MODERN USES OF THE WOLFBERRY

Building on ancient studies of the wolfberry, scientists in China today have conducted extensive research on the fruit's nutritional profile and health-promoting properties. These studies have added additional evidence that the wolfberry helps prevent free radical damage, supports a healthy immune system, improves vision and eye conditions, and assists in maintaining healthy blood sugar levels.

The Chinese Ministry of Public Health approved sales of the wolfberry as a botanical medicine in 1983, and the Chinese State Scientific and Technological commission has declared the wolfberry a "national treasure." Claims have been made that Olympic swimmers in China have benefited from the amazing properties of the wolfberry.

Health-promoting properties of the wolfberry include

- Prevents free radical damage
- Supports a healthy immune system
- Improves vision and eye conditions
- Assists in maintaining healthy blood sugar levels

FREE RADICAL DAMAGE

While everybody ages as part of the life process, excessive free radicals can accelerate the aging process at a cellular level. Free radicals are atoms with an odd or unpaired electron, and they can do damage at the fundamental DNA level in human cells. Dr. Bruce N. Ames, a researcher at UCLA, speculates that many cells in the human body are exposed to over one-hundred thousand free radical attacks each day. While the normal metabolic process generates free radicals, substances such as pesticides, tobacco smoke, environmental pollutants, and radiation can all significantly accelerate the production of free radicals in the body. Called the oxidation process, free radical damage to human cells is similar to the way metals become oxidized, resulting in rust.

Because free radical atoms have odd or unpaired electrons, they are in constant search of another electron to create a stable pair. When the free radical finds this electron, it creates a new free radical that is also missing an electron, which leads to a continuous process in which free radicals are regenerated. This is particularly damaging to cellular DNA, which leads to acceleration of the aging process.

A particularly damaging element of oxidation is the process of free radicals turning the lipids (fats) in the human body rancid. A brown waste product, lipofuscin, is created by this process, creating age spots on the hands, and interfering with synaptic communication in the brain. Lipofuscin deposits are also found in the liver, eyes, heart, and other organs. At age thirty, the amount of intracellular lipofuscin is about 35 percent; at age ninety, lipofuscin levels skyrocket to 78 percent.

In very simple terms, the process of free radical damage to DNA works like this:

- Free radicals attack thymine, one of the four nucleotide bases in DNA.
- As a result, thymadine glycol is formed.
- This oxidized thymadine's structure changes to a cluster.
- When DNA replicates, the cell attempts to repair the damaged part of the DNA by replacing it with new DNA.
- Numerous DNA repairs can lead to more cellular mutations.
- Cellular mutations can lead to malignant growth.

In a study conducted at Peking University in 2001, mitochondrial DNA deletion could actually be reduced by the introduction of wolfberry. Another study conducted in China found a 48 percent increase in super oxide dismutase and a 12 percent increase in hemoglobin in elderly study participants. The researchers also found a 65 percent decrease in serum lipid peroxidase, which indicates that the wolfberry is a potent antioxidant that may slow the aging process.

In addition, wolfberries contain powerful antioxidant flavonoids, the water-soluble plant pigments that give blueberries, peppers, oranges, and wolfberries their distinctive color. For the body to optimally utilize flavonoids, and the phytochemicals they contain, they should be consumed in whole foods like fruits and vegetables. A study conducted by Huang Yuanqing and colleagues at the Ningxia Medical College in Yinchuan, China, revealed that the total flavonoid constituents of *Lycium barbarum* have a significant inhibitory effect on the heat output of L_{1210} cells, producing a free radical scavenging effect.

According to the ORAC (oxygen radical absorbance capacity) test created at Tufts University, which measures a food's antioxidant properties, wolfberries top the list:

- Wolfberry juice   3,472
- Vitamin E oil   3,309
- Pomegranates   3,037
- Blueberries   2,400
- Noni fruit   1,506
- Raspberries   1,220

NUTRITIONAL PROPERTIES OF THE WOLFBERRY

The Beijing National Research Institute in 1988 conducted a study of the nutritional components of the wolfberry and found a true powerhouse. Wolfberries contain over 500 times more vitamin C than oranges, twenty-one trace minerals, eighteen amino acids, more beta-carotene than carrots, and more calcium than spinach. Eight ounces of wolfberries contains 4,000 RDA of vitamin B-1; 1,000 percent RDA of vitamin B-3; 190 percent RDA of fiber; and over 100 percent of the RDA for chromium, copper, iron, manganese, and potassium.

Beneficial nutritional and bioactive components of the wolfberry include:

- 500 times more vitamin C than oranges
- More beta-carotene than carrots
- 21 trace minerals
- 18 amino acids
- Essential fatty acids
- Over 1,000 percent of the RDA for two key B-vitamins
- More protein than whole wheat
- Solavetivone, a powerful antibacterial and antifungal agent
- Beta-sisterol, an anti-inflammatory agent
- Cyperone, a sesquiterpent that is beneficial for healthy blood pressure and heart function
- Physalin, with anticancer properties
- Betaine, which helps lower homocysteine levels that can contribute to heart disease

WOLFBERRIES CAN HELP SUPPORT A HEALTHY IMMUNE SYSTEM

Numerous studies have demonstrated that wolfberries support immune system functioning by increasing the lymphocyte transformation rate and improving the macrophage phagocytic function. Wolfberry increases T-cell immune response by increasing the number of E receptors on the surface of T cells or by increasing the numbers of T cells directly. One Chinese study showed that after taking wolfberry, lysozyme, IgG, and IgA in serum increased in all study participants. The activities of inter-leukin 2 (IL-2) increased by 226 percent in two-thirds of the participants. In another study, eating wolfberries strengthened immunoglobulin A levels (an index of immune function).

WOLFBERRIES CAN HELP IMPROVE VISION

Both ancient wisdom and modern scientific studies have demonstrated that wolfberries are beneficial for improving vision. One study tested the effects of the wolfberry on the eyesight of twenty-seven subjects. Dark adaptation dramatically improved, physiologic scotoma decreased, and serum vitamin A and carotene content increased—all of which are indicators of eyesight acuity. Also, the pigments lutein and zeaxanthin, both of which are contained in wolfberries, have been demonstrated to protect the retina by neutralizing the free radicals from sunlight that may damage eye tissue.

WOLFBERRIES CAN ASSIST IN MAINTAINING HEALTHY BLOOD SUGAR LEVELS

Among the wolfberry's other health-promoting proper-ties, studies have demonstrated that it also has a benefi-cial effect on blood sugar levels and can be of possible benefit to those suffering from diabetes and pre-diabetic conditions.

Qiong Luo and collaborators at the University of Hong Kong and Wuhan University, in a study of the wolfberry's glucose stabilizing properties, said, "It was found that the three *Lycium barbarum* fruit extracts/fractions could sig-nificantly reduce blood glucose levels and serum total cho-lesterol (TC) and triglyceride (TG) concentrations and at same time markedly increase high density lipoprotein cholesterol (HDL-c) levels after ten days treatment in test-ed rabbits, indicating that there were substantial hypo-glycemic and hypolipidemic effects.

"Hypoglycemic effect of LBP-X was more significant than those of water decoction and crude LBP, but its hypolipidemic effect seemed to be weaker. Total antioxi-dant capacity assay showed that all three *Lycium barbarum* extracts/fractions possessed antioxidant activity."

HOW TO USE WOLFBERRIES

- Chew 1/2 to 1 ounce of wolfberries each morning and evening.
- Brew a tea with 3/4 ounce of wolfberries and drink every day.

- Mix 1/2 to 1 ounce of wolfberries with cereal to make a healthy breakfast.
- Use wolfberries just like raisins in muffins and breads.

WHY IT'S HOT!

The wolfberry, ancient China's "national treasure" that has bestowed youth and vigor on generations of Chinese, is now available as modern America's most potent anti-oxidant food. Numerous clinical studies have demonstrated that the wolfberry can play a significant role in preventing free radical damage and oxidative stress, supporting a healthy immune system, improving vision, and assisting in maintaining healthy blood sugar levels.

This simple berry that tastes of cranberries and cherries is also a nutritional powerhouse with more vitamin C than oranges, more beta-carotene than carrots, and more protein than whole wheat. In fact, some have said that the wolfberry comes as close as any other food to a multi-vitamin. So chew an ounce of wolfberries in the morning, brew some wolfberry tea, and make some wolfberry muffins—and reap the healthful benefits of these amazing berries.

REFERENCES

"African Plant May Help Fight Fat," CBS News' *60 Minutes*, November 23, 2004.

"The Anti-Fat Pill and the Bushmen," ABC TV, August 25, 2003.

Ahima, R.S. & Osei, S.Y., "Molecular regulation of eating behavior: new insights and prospects for therapeutic strategies," Trends Mol Med, 7, 205–13 (2001).

Alpha-mangostin-induced apoptosis in human leukemia HL60 cells. http://www.ncbi.nlm.nih.gov/entrez/query.fcgi?cmd=Retrieve&db=PubMed&list_uids=15498656&dopt=Citation.

Anderson R.A., Broadhurst C.L., Polansky M.M., Schmidt W.F., Khan A., Flanagan V.P., Schoene N.W., Graves D.J. "Isolation and characterization of polyphenol type-A polymers from cinnamon with insulin-like biological activity." Diabetes Res Clin Pract. 2003 Dec; 62(3): 139–48.

Anthocyanins and Flavonoids. http://www.polyphenols.com/background.htm.

Antibacterial activity of xanthones. http://www.ncbi.nlm.nih.gov/entrez/query.fcgi?cmd=Retrieve&db=PubMed&list_uids=8887739&dopt=Abstract.

Ben Cao Gang Mu (Ming Dynasty 1368–1644 A.D.) People's Health Publishing Press, 1982, Chinese version translated by Sue Chao.

Beta-carotene as an antioxidant. http://www.jacn.org/cgi/content/full/18/5/426.

Blumenthal, Mark *Herbal Medicine: Expanded Edition E Monographs*, Lippincott Williams & Wilkins, 2000.

Bouchard C., Perusse L., "Genetic aspects of obesity," Annals of the New York Academy of Sciences, 1993; 699: 26–35.

Broadhurst C.L., Polansky M.M., Anderson R.A. "Insulin-like biological activity of culinary and medicinal plant aqueous extracts in vitro." J Agric Food Chem 2000 Mar; 48(3): 849–52.

Calucci L., Pinzino C., Zandomeneghi M., et al. "Effects of gamma-irradiation on the free radical and antioxidant contents in nine aromatic herbs and spices." J Agric Food Chem 2003 Feb 12; 51(4): 927–34.

Cao GW, Yang WG, Du P. Observation of the Effects of LAK/IL–2 Therapy Combined with Lycium Barbarum Polysaccharides in the Treatment of 75 Cancer Patients. Chunghua Chung Liu Tsa Chih. 1994, Nov.; 16(6): 428–431.

Cheng et al. Fasting Plasma zeaxanthin Response to Fructus Barbarum L. (Wolfberry; Kei Tze) in a Food-based human Supplementation Trial. British Journal of Nutrition (2005), 93, 123–130.

Components of mangosteen. http://www.ars-grin.gov/cgi-bin/duke/farmacy2.pl?1228.

Ding Aurong, Li Shuli. Effects on Activities of Na+, K+-ATP Enzymes from Huang Jing and Five Other Herbs. Zhong Cheng Yao (Chinese Patent Herbs). 1990, (9): 28.

Ensminger A.H., Esminger M.K.J., et al. *Food for Health: A Nutrition Encyclopedia.* Clovis, California: Pegus Press, 1986.

Epicatechins. http://www.worldofmolecules.com/antioxidants/epicatechin.htm.

Food navigator alert. "Fruit Antioxidant, the next cholesterol-lowering ingredient?"

Fortin, François, Editorial Director. *The Visual Foods Encyclopedia.* Macmillan, New York.

Free radicals and aging. http://www.physics.ohio-state.edu/~ wilkins/writing/Samples/shortmed/nelson/radicals.html.

Free radicals. http://www.exrx.net/Nutrition/Antioxidants/Introduction.html.

Fujita, M. et al. "Purification and characterization of a strong fibrinolytic enzyme (nattokinase) in the vegetable cheese natto, a popular soybean fermented food in Japan." Biochem Biophys Res Commun 1993; 30: 1340–47.

Geng Changshan, Wang Geying, Lin Yongdong, et al. Effects on Mouse Lymphocyte and T Cells from Lycium Barbarum Polysaccharide (LBP). Zhong Cao Yao (Chinese Herbs). 1988,19(7):25.

Grieve M. *A Modern Herbal.* Dover Publications, New York.

Habeck, Martina, "A succulent cure to end obesity," Drug Discovery Today, 2002 Mar 1; 7(5): 280–81. Tulp, Orien Lee; Harbi, Nevin A. 2002. "Hoodia species as a source of essential micronutrients." FASEB Journal, Vol. 16 NO. 4 March 20, 2002 PP. A654.

Hager, K. et al. "Fibrinogen and Aging." Again (Milano) 1994, 6: 133–38.

Harkins, K., 2000. "What's the use of cranberry juice?" Age and Ageing, 29: 9–12.

He Jie, Pan Li, Guo Fuxiang, et al. Hepatoprotective Effects from Lycium Barbarum Fruit in a Mouse Experiment. China Pharmacology and Toxicology. 1993, 7(4): 293.

Health Sciences Institute. "Prevent heart attack and stroke with potent enzyme that dissolves deadly blood clots in hours." March 2002.

Heinrich, J. et al. "Fibrinogen and factor VII in the prediction of coronary risk." Arterioscler Thromb 1994, 14: 54–59.

http://en.wikipedia.org/wiki/Tibetan_Goji_berry

http://worldshealthiestfoods.com/sitesearch.php?sstr=cranberry&how=1&x=0&y=0.

http://www.cranberryinstitue.org/health/bibliography.htm.

http://www.foodnavigator.com/news/preintNewsBis.asp?id=54316.

http://www.nutraingredients-usa.com/news/printNewsBis. asp?id=63231.

http://www.wholehealthmd.com/print/view/1,1560,SU_782,00.htm.

Huang Di Nei Jing (*Yellow Emperor's Classic of Internal Medicine*) Chinese medical textbook dating to the Qin and Han periods (221 B.C.–220 A.D.). Tianjin Scientific Technology Publishing Press, 1986. Chinese version translated by research scientist Sue Chao.

Huang Guifang, Luo Jieying. Immune Boosting Effects from Fu Fang Wu Zi Yang Zong Wan (a Chinese patent herb containing Lycium barbarum fruit). Zhong Cao Yao (Chinese Herbs). 1990, 12(6): 27.

Hydrogen peroxide.http://www.thedoctorslounge.net/medlounge/articles/freeradicals/freeradicals5.htm.

Impari-Radosevich J., Deas S., Polansky M.M., et al. "Regulation of PTP-1 and insulin receptor kinase by fractions from cinnamon: implications for cinnamon regulation of insulin signaling." Horm Res 1998 Sep; 50(3): 177–82.

Khan A., Safdar M., Ali Khan M.M., Khattak K.N., Anderson R.A. "Cinnamon improves glucose and lipids of people with type 2 diabetes." Diabetes Care. 2003 Dec; 26(12): 3215–18.

Kim H.P., Kim S.Y., Lee E.J., Kim Y.C. Zeaxanthin Dipalmitate from Lycium Barbarum Has Hepatoprotective Activity. Res. Commun Mol Pathol Pharmacol. 1997, Sep.; (3): 301–314.

LDL oxidation inhibition by xanthones. http://www.ncbi.nlm.nih.gov/entrez/query.fcgi?cmd=Retrieve&db=PubMed&list_uids=11200095&dopt=Abstract.

Leahy, M., 2002. "Latest Developments in Cranberry Health Research." Pharma Biol, 40 (Suppl): 50–54.

Lee, Deborah. *Essential Fatty Acids*. Pleasant Grove, UT: Woodland Publishing, 1997.

Li Wei, Dai Shouzhi, Ma Fu, et al. Active Lymphocyte Effects Observed after Taking Lycium Barbarum Fruits. Zhong Cao Yao (Chinese Herbs). 1991, 22(6): 251.

Li yuhao, Deng Xiangchao, Wu Heqing, et al. The Effect on Lipid Metabolism of Injured Liver Cells in Rat. Zhong Guo Zhong Yao Za Zhi (Journal of Chinese Herbal Medicine). 1994, 19(5):300.

Lipid peroxidation and xanthones. http://www.ncbi.nlm.nih.gov/entrez/query.fcgi?cmd=Retrieve&db=PubMed&list_uids=11200095&dopt=Abstract.

Lu CX, Cheng BQ. Radiosensitizing Effects of Lycium Barbarum Polysaccharide of Lewis Lung Cancer. Chung His I chieh Ho Tsa Chih. 1991, Oct.: 11(10): 611–612.

Lycium barbarum Medical Effects, improves eyesight, Ningxia Scientific and Technological Commission, July 1982–Jan. 1984.

MacLean D.B., Luo L-G. "Increased ATP content/production in the hypothalamus may be a signal for energy sensing of satiety: studies of the anorectic mechanism of a plant steroidal glycoside." Brain Res 2004; 1020: 1–11.

http://www.crfg.org/pubs/ff/mango.html.

Mangold, Tom, "Sampling the Kalahari cactus diet," BBC2 News, May 30, 2003.

http://gears.tucson.ars.ag.gov/book/chap5/mangosteen.html.

http://hort.purdue.edu/newcrop/morton/mangosteen.html.

http://hort.purdue.edu/newcrop/morton/mangosteen.html.

Maruyama M., Sumi H., "Effect of Natto diet on blood pressure." JTTAS, 1995.

Montalescot, G. et al. "Fibrinogen as a risk factor for coronary heart disease." Eur Heart J 1998, 19 Suppl H:H11–17.

Mosby's Handbook of Herbs and Supplements and Their Therapeutic Uses. St. Louis: Elsevier Science, 2003.

Murcia M.A., Egea I., Romojaro F., Parras P., Jimenez A.M., Martinez-Tome M. "Antioxidant evaluation in dessert spices compared with common food additives. Influence of irradiation procedure." J Agric Food Chem. 2004 Apr 7; 52(7): 1872–81.

National Center for Health Statistics, Centers for Disease Control. Prevalence of Overweight among Children and Adolescents: United States, 1999.

Natural Medicine's Comprehensive Database, Therapeutic Research Facility, Stockton, Calif., 2002.

Nishimura K, Hamamoto J, Adachi K, Yamazaki A, Takagi S., Tamai T. "Natto diet was apparently effective in a case of incipient central retinal vein occlusion." Jpn Rev Clin Ophthalmol.1994; Sept 88(9): 1381–85.

Nursing Herbal Medicine Handbook, 2001.

Otsuka H., Fujioka S., Komiya T., et al. "Studies on anti-inflammatory agents;" "Anti-inflammatory constituents of Cinnamomum sieboldii Meissn." Yakugaku Zasshi 1982 Jan; 102(2): 162–72.

Ouattara B., Simard R.E., Holley R.A., et al. "Antibacterial activity of selected fatty acids and essential oils against six meat spoilage organisms." Int J Food Microbiol 1997 Jul 22; 37(2–3): 155–62.

PDR for Herbal Medicines. Montvale, N.J: Thomson PDR, 2004.

Peirce, Andrea *The American Pharmaceutical Association's Practical Guide to Natural Medicines,* 1999.

Phenolic compounds and oxidative stress. http://www.bio.puc.cl/vinsalud/publica/biolresrevision.doc.

Physicians' Desk Reference for Nutritional Supplements. Montvale, N.J.: Thomson PDR, 2001.

PubMed—antituberculosis research. http://www.ncbi.nlm.nih.gov/entrez/query.fcgi?cmd=Retrieve&db=PubMed&list_uids=12843596&dopt=Abstract.

PubMed—histaminergic and serotonergic blocking agent. http://www.ncbi.nlm.nih.gov/entrez/query.fcgi?cmd=Retrieve&db=PubMed&list_uids=8923814&dopt=Abstract.

PubMed—leukemia research. http://www.ncbi.nlm.nih.gov/entrez/query.fcgi?cmd=Retrieve&db=PubMed&list_uids=12932141&dopt=Abstract.

PubMed—liver cancer research. http://www.ncbi.nlm.nih.gov/entrez/query.fcgi?cmd=Retrieve&db=PubMed&list_uids=12451486&dopt=Abstract.

Qi Zongshao, Li Shufang, Wu Jiping, et al. Chemical Analysis on Lycium Barbarum Fruit and Leaves. Zhong Yao Tong Bao (Chinese Herb News). 1986, 11(3):41.

Qin B., Nagasaki M., Ren M., Bajotto G., Oshida Y., Sato Y. "Cinnamon extract prevents the insulin resistance induced by a high-fructose diet." Horm Metab Res. 2004 Feb; 36(2): 119–25.

Qin B., Nagasaki M., Ren M., Bajotto G., Oshida Y., Sato Y. "Cinnamon extract (traditional herb) potentiates in vivo insulin-regulated glucose utilization via enhancing insulin signaling in rats." Diabetes Res Clin Pract. 2003 Dec; 62(3): 139–48.

Quale J.M., Landman D., Zaman M.M., et al. "In vitro activity of Cinnamomum zeylanicum against azole resistant and sensitive Candida species and a pilot study of cinnamon for oral candidiasis." Am J Chin Med 1996; 24(2): 103–09.

Scalbert, A., et al., 2005. "Polyphenols: antioxidants and beyond." Am J Clin Nutr, 81(Suppl): 215S–7S.

Serdula, M.K., Ivery, D., Coates, R.J., et al., "Do obese children become obese adults? A review of the literature," Preventive Medicine, 1993; 22: 167–77.

State Scientific and Technological Commission of China, Clinical Experiment on Lycium, Register No. 870306.

State Scientific and Technological Commission of China, Pharmacological Experiment on Lycium, Register No. 870303.

Sumi H. "Healthy microbe 'bacillus natto.'" Japan Bio Science Laboratory Co. Ltd.

Sumi H. Interview with Doctor of Medicine Hiroyuki Sumi. Japan Bio Science Laboratory Co. Ltd. 9. Sumi H. "Structure and Fibrinolytic Properties of Nattokinase."

Sumi H., Hamada H., Mihara H. "A novel strong fibrinolytic enzyme (nattokinase) in the vegetable cheese 'natto.'" International 5. Journal of Fibronolysis and Thrombolysis. Abstracts of the ninth international congress on fibrinolysis, Amsterdam, 1988, Vol.2, Sup.1: 67.

Sumi H., Hamada H., Nakanishi K., Hiratani H. "Enhancement of the fibrinolytic activity in plasma by oral administration of nattokinase." Acta Haematol 1990; 84(3): 139–43.

Takenaga M., Hirai A., Terano T., et al. "In vitro effect of cinnamic aldehyde, a main component of Cinnamomi Cortex, on human platelet aggregation and arachidonic acid metabolism." J Pharmacobiodyn 1987 May; 10 (5): 201–08.

Tannins. http://www.ansci.cornell.edu/plants/toxicagents/tannin/

Tao Maoxuan, Zhao Zhongliang. In Vitro Anti-Mutation Effect of Lycium Barbarum Polysaccharide (LBP). Zong Cao Yao (Chinese Herbs). 1992, 23(9):474.

The Cranberry Institute: Emerging Research: http://www.cranberryinstitue.org/emerging.htm.

Thompson G., "Bushmen squeeze money from a humble cactus," *The New York Times*, April 1, 2003.

Tulp O.L., Harbi N.A., Mihalov J., DerMarderosian A., "Effect of Hoodia plant on food intake and body weight in lean and obese LA/Ntul//-cp rats," FASEB Journal, March 7, 2001, Vol. 15 No. 4, A404.

Tulp, Orien Lee; Harbi, Nevin A.; DerMarderosian, Ara, "Effect of Hoodia plant on weight loss in congenic obese LA/Ntul//-cp rats." FASEB Journal, March 20, 2002, Vol. 16 NO. 4, A648.

Understanding Free Radicals and Antioxidants. http://www.health checksystems.com/antioxid.htm.

Van Heerden F.R., Vleggaar R., Horak R.M., Learmonth R.A., Maharaj V., Whittal R.D., "Pharmaceutical compositions having appetite suppression activity," United States Patent 6,376,657, issued April 23, 2002.

VanderEnde D.S., Morrow J.D. "Release of markedly increased quantities of prostaglandin D2 from the skin in vivo in humans after the application of cinnamic aldehyde." J Am Acad Dermatol 2001 Jul; 45(1): 62–67.

Wang Qiang, Chen Suiqing, Zhang Zhehua, et al. The Measurement of Lycium Barbarum Polysaccharide (LBP) in Lycium Barbarum Fruit. Zhong Cao Yao (Chinese Herbs). 1991, 22(2):67.

Weil, Andrew, M.D. *Eating Well for Optimum Health: The Essential Guide to Food, Diet, and Nutrition.* New York: Knopf, 2000.

Whitaker, R.C., Wright, J.A., Pepe, M.S., Seidel, K.D., Dietz, W.H., "Predicting obesity in young adulthood from childhood and parental obesity," New England Journal of Medicine, 1997; 337: 869–73.

Wikipedia free-content on-line encyclopedia http://en.wikipedia. org/wiki/Natto.

Wood, Rebecca. The Whole Foods Encyclopedia. New York, NY: Prentice-Hall Press; 1988.

www.1stchinese herbs.com/lycium_fruit.

www.berryyoungjuice.com/brief.jsp.

www.naturalhealthway.com/wolfberry/wolfberrystudies.

www.rawfood.com.

www.webdeb.com/oils/wolfberries.

Xanthone and Human Leukemia cells. www.ncbi.nlm.nih.gov/ entrez/query.fcgi?cmd=Retrieve&db=PubMed&list_uids=1293 2141&dopt=Citation.

Xanthones. http://www.biocyc.org/META/new-image?object= XANTHONE-SYN.

Xiaojun Y., et al., 2002. "Antioxidant Activities and Antitumor Screening of Extracts from Cranberry Fruit." J Agric Food Chem, 50(21): 5844–49.

Zhong Guo Shipin Bao (China Food News). March 2, 1998

Zoladz P., Raudenbush B., Lilley S. "Cinnamon perks performance." Paper presented at the annual meeting of the Association for Chemoreception Sciences, held in Sarasota, FL, April 21–25, 2004.